# EASY
# PERIMENOPAUSE

The Essential Guide to Modern Midlife

JENNIFER WOODWARD

MS | FDNP

**Finesse**

To my family –
Beau, Jackson, Rebecca Sky,
Roman, and Chase.

And to every woman in midlife
looking for guidance and support.

# Table of Contents

## CHAPTER 1

# Welcome to Perimenopause – You're Not Alone

Did you know that nine out of ten women have never been taught about perimenopause (1)? This means that 90% of women entering midlife suddenly experience mood swings, weight gain, insomnia, and fatigue, without any idea of what's really happening to them.

If you're like most women, you'll first try to manage the symptoms on your own. Then, you'll probably go to your doctor or OB/GYN for an explanation and some relief. Since there's no diagnosis for perimenopause and no one drug that will resolve all the symptoms you're experiencing, you'll probably be told *your lab work is normal*. Or *you're just getting older*. Or my personal favorite: *it's all in your head*.

As a functional health practitioner with a Master's in Integrative Nutrition, my work with perimenopausal women over nearly a decade has taught me that women's symptoms are *not* in their heads. Studies have shown that during the perimenopause transition, 79% of women suffer from hot flashes, 75% start experiencing erratic menstrual cycles, and 71% complain of worsening cognitive issues and brain fog.

A total of 51% of women report dealing with anxiety, 38% experience sleep difficulties, and 28% struggle with depression. These symptoms are so bothersome that nearly 90% of women in the perimenopause transition seek out advice from their doctor on how to cope with these problems (1, 2, 3, 4).

If you're suddenly experiencing any of these (or other) confusing symptoms, you might be in perimenopause. But don't worry—you're not alone, and you've come to the right place. In this chapter, I will validate your experiences and begin to equip you with essential knowledge about your symptoms so that you know exactly how to start feeling better, ASAP.

## What Is Perimenopause and How Do I Know If I'm Experiencing It?

**Perimenopause** is the transition to menopause. It is marked by changes in menstrual flow and the length of the cycle due to sudden surges in estrogen (1). During the perimenopause transition, symptoms may include:

- Hot flashes
- Vaginal and sexual changes
- Sleep problems
- Anxiety
- Weight gain (especially around the belly)
- Depression
- Rage
- Itchiness
- Gut issues
- Food sensitivities
- Decreased libido

• Changing menstrual patterns

*If you have three or more of these symptoms, congratulations! You're likely in perimenopause.*

At this point in your journey, you may not be educated on perimenopause. But you're certainly savvy! You know that the changes you are experiencing in your period, sleep, energy, mood, and weight are challenging, and they're definitely not in your head. But maybe you're unsure of what to do about these symptoms.

Your doctor might have offered you "the pill" for your heavy periods, an antidepressant for your mood swings, and a weight loss shot for the few extra pounds around your waist. But you know there's something else going on. And if you're like most women reading this book, you don't want to take a drug to address it. That's how I felt, too.

# My Story

I was the firstborn in a family of three girls, and I was pushed to perform my best throughout grade school and high school. In my extremely structured life, year-round sports, extra-curricular activities, and honors classes were the norm. The pressure of trying to appear perfect came with a price: I started secretly binging on large quantities of junk food that were hidden around my house.

Always a bit on the chubbier side, I started noticeably gaining weight. Until one summer when my grandfather offered me twenty dollars to lose twenty pounds. As a family member regularly made remarks about my "pregnant belly," telling me to "suck it in," I took on the challenge of getting fit.

I spent the summer before my junior year of high school drinking gallons of artificially flavored water, eating very little, and working out with a neighbor for two hours each day. At the end of the summer, I was rewarded with a new, slimmer body along with a growth spurt; I shot up from 5'5" to 5'11" in just over three months.

But my new physique came with a price. Previously blissfully oblivious to the world of dieting, I became obsessed with calories, fat, sugar, and exercise. In high school, I woke up early enough to fit in a workout for one hour before my classes, finishing my school day with another two hours of track, soccer, or volleyball practice. Weekends were spent drinking too much alcohol and throwing up the fast food I would inevitably binge on after cheap vodka lowered my inhibitions and forced me to realize how hungry I truly was.

College at the University of California at Davis brought more of the same—high academic performance, early graduation, working multiple jobs at once, restricting food (and consequently binging and purging), excessive partying, and compulsive exercise. I was also long-distance dating the love of my life, Beau Woodward. Anyone who's dated long-distance knows how stressful it can be!

At the beginning of my sophomore year of college, I moved back home and married Beau. After graduating and spending a few years in the workforce as a pharmaceutical sales rep for Abbott Labs, I had four children with Beau in a very short time. My desire to look perfect on the outside grew stronger with each passing year. Diet and exercise routines were obsessively structured as I fought hard to "get my body back" after each pregnancy, even though I carried an extra twenty to thirty pounds in between babies. Restricting calories led to food and alcohol binges. My sleep was poor, my nutrition was worse, and my stress management was non-existent. In fact, I actually believed that I thrived on stress.

It wasn't long before my health hit rock bottom. After the birth of our third child, I started experiencing insomnia and panic attacks. Each morning, I felt so tired that it was almost impossible to drag myself out of bed. The three cups of coffee I would drink on an empty stomach didn't do much to help my exhaustion.

I couldn't lose my pregnancy weight, even though I was doing two workouts a day and following a very low-carbohydrate diet. My stomach pudge was spilling over my yoga pants, my hair was falling out, and my nails were splitting and peeling. My stomach was a mess. I only pooped once a week and I was constantly bloated, despite only eating "clean" foods. My moods were all over the place, and my PMS and period symptoms seemed to worsen with every passing month.

I needed help, so I went to my doctor. He offered me Prozac for my mood swings and the birth control pill for my period issues. I looked at the doctor I trusted, genuinely confused. I wasn't depressed and I wasn't trying to prevent pregnancy, so the medications seemed useless. I left the office feeling hopeless. I went back to scouring the internet, praying to find information that would help me.

One winter night—sleepless and sweaty as usual—I found a video online that changed everything. The woman in the video called herself a Functional Diagnostic Nutrition Practitioner (FDNP)©, and she was sharing information about the lab testing that she ran on her clients. I had never heard of these labs, which looked for imbalances in the hormone, digestive, and nervous systems. This woman's clients seemed to suffer from many of the symptoms I was dealing with. And it looked like they were experiencing relief, quickly.

Being a driven, Type A kind of girl, I didn't want to be a *client*. I wanted to be a *practitioner*. So, I signed up to pursue my certification as an FDNP. As part of the program, I was able to run all of the lab tests on myself with the help and guidance of experienced mentors and clinicians. We found multiple shocking imbalances in my labs. I had the hormones of a postmenopausal woman, my stress hormones were tanked, I had multiple bacterial and parasite infections in my gut, and I was sensitive to many of the foods I ate on a daily basis. I thought I was the healthiest person I knew, and I went through a short period of depression, realizing the seemingly healthy things I was doing weren't actually healthy at all! Low-carb diets, heavy workouts, and skimping on sleep to maximize productivity were only a few of the habits that I would have to change.

Using the protocols I was taught, I systematically addressed each issue and quickly found myself starting to feel better. Sleep became a friend once again, my weight normalized, and my mood was balanced enough that my husband was actually enjoying my company.

My friends began to notice my newfound health, and they wanted access to the same information. So I went into business of helping other perimenopausal women.

As I started to work with more people, my cases got more difficult and I recognized that I needed more education. I went back to school to get my master's in integrative nutrition.

Since I loved functional diagnostic nutrition (FDN) education so much, I began working for the FDN Certification

Program, managing their graduate association while building and running their business school. To learn everything I possibly could about women's health and hormones, I took on any independent contract work I could for other doctors and practitioners.

And now I want to share that information with you. *The consensus among my friends and clients is that, for most women, the general lack of education on perimenopause is frustrating and confusing.*

It's my goal to cut through the confusion and empower you to care for yourself well. As British author Trisha Posner writes in her book, *This is Not Your Mother's Menopause: One Woman's Natural Journey Through the Change*, "Our mothers were largely silent about what happened to them as they passed through this midlife change. But a new generation of women has already started to break the wall of silence" (5). That's us, sister! Together, we are breaking that wall of silence.

In this book, you'll meet a lot of the women I work with in my private practice. These women represent so many of us at this stage in life. Many of my clients are Type A perfectionists. They're driven. They excel at being moms, wives, employees, and employers. They can handle a lot at once. But perimenopause has thrown them for a loop. You'll learn about the steps I take as an FDN practitioner to help these women take back control of their lives. And you'll learn how to implement these steps so you can start feeling your very best too—even as you navigate perimenopause.

# Meet Your Perimenopausal Sisters

## *Elisa*

Every morning when Elisa opened her eyes, her stomach already felt tender and bloated. She had to drag herself out of bed to take care of her two young daughters while working two jobs. It had been years since she'd had a good night's sleep.

Elisa knew that exercise was supposed to be good for her, but every time she tried to work out, she experienced fatigue that lasted for days. Eventually, she noticed that she gained weight every time she worked out and had to quit exercising completely. Even though she barely ate, the pounds kept piling on In fact, she was rarely hungry. The smell of food made her nauseous, and she avoided many foods altogether because she just didn't have an appetite.

Being from the beautiful state of Texas, Elisa loved the outdoors. But spending too much time in the sun gave her symptoms similar to heatstroke. She passed out at the zoo one afternoon while walking around with her daughters. This terrified her. She was worried that she would lose consciousness again and wouldn't be able to care for her children.

## *Jenna*

Jenna loved her dual roles as a mom and teacher. Spending her days in a classroom and running carpool by late afternoon, she needed plenty of energy to keep up with the demands of daily life.

But she was dragging. Her energy was so low that, by the time she got to her day off each Thursday, she needed an entire day to rest and recover from the toll of the previous three days. She would wake up and put on a happy face as she got her kids out the door for school. Then she would sink straight into her plush linen couch, grimacing at the specks of dust on the coffee table but lacking the energy to do anything about it.

And she was gaining weight. Jenna could feel the full twenty pounds she had put on over the last year. She hated not being able to fit into her clothes. No stranger to dieting, she had spent years on popular eating plans like Weight Watchers and Atkins.

After years of hormonal problems, she had a hysterectomy at the young age of 39. She also suffered from Hashimoto's thyroiditis. Jenna knew deep down that if something didn't change in her life, she'd end up with even bigger health problems.

## *Tasha*

Tasha hadn't felt like herself in years. Formerly active and fit, she now worked from home and sat in front of her computer all day. Many times throughout her work day, she would wistfully glance at the gleaming Peloton bike gathering dust in her living room. She and her husband had just relocated from the suburbs to a big city and she felt out of sorts. Her husband worked nights, so Tasha often found herself alone.

Depression set in, and feelings of anxiety started to plague her regularly. When I met with her for the first time, Tasha reported that she was struggling with the following frustrations:

*"The monthly hormonal highs and lows are becoming more extreme. I have at least one week of extremely sad, crying days. This completely derails me and kicks me off my fitness path and is now interrupting my performance at work. No matter how much activity I add to my routine, I continue*

*to gain weight. I feel better exercising, but the weight stays. And if I do lose anything, it is small and insignificant and eventually comes back. It even increases."*

Tasha noticed that her weight gain started after she had her gallbladder removed. She knew that her regular indulgence in alcohol and pasta, inadequate sleep, and lack of consistent exercise compounded her feelings of depression and moodiness. Doctors had provided no real help, so Tasha set out to heal herself naturally.

Elisa, Jenna, and Tasha are real women. The symptoms of perimenopause crept up on each of them slowly, derailing their efforts to care for themselves. Weight gain, insomnia, brain fog, mood swings, and period problems were just a few of the frustrating symptoms these women were battling. You're going to hear more about them throughout this book, but you'll be pleased to know they overcame their struggles, naturally. And you can too!

First, you have to understand why your symptoms have gotten so bad in the first place. Let me introduce you to **the Overs**.

## The Overs

I work with women in midlife every single day, and I'm seeing them enter perimenopause earlier than ever. In fact, most of my clients begin to experience symptoms as early as their mid-thirties.

*Why is this?*

My theory is that Western women today are *chronically stuck in fight-or-flight mode* due to **the Overs:**

- Over-dieting
- Over-exercising
- Over-stressing
- Being over-tired

# What Is Fight-or-Flight Mode?

The autonomic nervous system consists of two main parts that govern the body's automatic processes: the **sympathetic nervous system** and the **parasympathetic nervous system**. The sympathetic system is associated with the **fight-or-flight response**, while the parasympathetic system is referred to as the **rest-and-digest response**. The balance between these two systems is called homeostasis.

These two systems work together to balance the processes of the body. For example, the heart receives signals from both the sympathetic and parasympathetic systems. One cue signals the heart rate to increase, and the other tells the heart rate to decrease. Thankfully, we don't have to think about regulating our own heart rate; the autonomic nervous system does it for us.

The average woman tends to cultivate a lifestyle that keeps her in the fight-or-flight response for most of the day. She wakes up early, often to work out on an empty stomach. She skips breakfast and drinks coffee during the morning. She eats a light lunch or sometimes skips lunch entirely, preferring to snack instead. She finishes her morning and afternoon duties at work or at home in time to pick up the kids and run them around for afternoon and evening activities. Dinner is an afterthought, and often fast food becomes a substitute for a nourishing meal. By the time she actually gets home in the evening, the only thing she wants is a giant glass of wine. She'll snack on popcorn or chips to unwind. She stays up after the kids go to bed for some much needed "me time," watching TV or scrolling on her phone before trying to get to bed around midnight. She can't really fall or stay asleep, and she dreads the day to come when she has to do it all over again.

*Does this sound like you? This is the plight of women everywhere.* Each part of the day keeps women in a state of chronic fight-or-flight. The sympathetic nervous system is continually activated as the stress hormone **cortisol** floods the system throughout the day.

# Fight-or-Flight Mode and the Cortisol Problem

**Cortisol** is a hormone that our adrenal glands produce when we're stressed or our blood sugar is low. It regulates how our body responds to stress, reduces inflammation, and assists in memory formulation.

Both cortisol and the sympathetic nervous system are closely interconnected as part of the body's response to stress. When we encounter a stressful situation, the sympathetic nervous system kicks in and triggers the fight-or-flight response, causing the release of cortisol and other hormones. By increasing our energy levels and keeping us alert, cortisol helps us cope during such stressful times.

This would normally be a helpful survival mechanism for our beautifully designed bodies. Historically, humans have effortlessly cycled into and out of fight-or-flight mode. When we experienced true stressors (like hunger, danger, or cold), the sympathetic nervous system kicked in to release cortisol and bolster our ability to deal with them. Stressors were generally acute and transient, which allowed the body to quickly release the hormones needed to adapt to the danger for a short period.

Stress isn't inherently bad. As we have already discussed, there are good stressors that enable our bodies to evolve and adapt. But historically, a stressor would come and then go. Our ancestors probably only went into fight-or-flight mode during life-threatening situations.

Today, most women rarely experience truly life-threatening situations. However, we do give our bodies the signal that danger is imminent and prolonged. By **over-dieting, overstressing, overexercising,** and being **overtired**, we tell our bodies that we are constantly in danger. In response, our bodies constantly activate fight-or-flight mode.

Why is this a problem? *Chronic stress can disrupt the natural balance of hormones in the body, leading to mood swings, weight gain, insomnia, and fatigue.* Moreover, cortisol levels that are elevated over a prolonged period can weaken the immune system and increase the risk of heart disease and other health complications. Chronic stress can also lead to high levels of internal inflammation.

## Inflammation

Inflammation is the body's natural response to injury or infection, a protective effort involving immune cells, blood vessels, and molecules that eliminate the problem and start the healing process. This process begins when tissues are injured by bacteria, trauma, toxins, heat, or any other cause. The damaged cells release chemicals like histamine, bradykinin, and prostaglandins. These substances cause blood vessels to leak fluid into the tissues, resulting in swelling. This swelling helps separate the foreign substance from further contact with body tissues (6).

Inflammation triggers a series of events within the immune system. White blood cells are mobilized to the site of injury or infection, where they engulf and consume foreign substances. The process of inflammation is characterized by signs like redness, warmth, swelling, and pain. While acute inflammation is essential for healing, chronic inflammation can contribute to various diseases, including some types of cancer, rheumatoid arthritis, atherosclerosis, and hormone imbalance.

Women in perimenopause tend to suffer from increasing levels of inflammation. This inflammation may show up in the form of:

- Headaches
- Brain fog
- Skin issues like acne and eczema
- Joint pain
- Swelling and water retention
- Increasingly heavy periods
- Weight gain
- Anxiety
- Depression

Elevated cortisol levels can also worsen inflammation in the body. As a steroid hormone, cortisol itself is anti-inflammatory by nature. However, long-term exposure to high levels of cortisol in the bloodstream can lead to muscle and organ tissue breakdown. It can also increase **inflammatory cytokines**, which are signaling molecules that are produced by immune cells and other cell types to promote inflammation. While inflammation is a normal part of the body's response to injury, it can become harmful if it occurs in healthy tissues or goes on for too long.

Chronic inflammation can also prevent healing (7). The body requires hormonal balance to repair and regenerate tissues, regulate bodily functions, and maintain overall well-being. When the body remains in a continuous state of stress, the healing processes that rely on hormonal regulation are compromised. This makes it difficult for the body to heal itself effectively.

## Restoration and the Parasympathetic Nervous System

**Restoration** is what we're after, especially in perimenopause. *The antidote to fight-or-flight mode is to spend more time in the parasympathetic state of the autonomic nervous system.* When the body is at rest or in a non-stressful situation, the parasympathetic nervous system takes over. It helps our bodies conserve energy by:

- Slowing the heart rate
- Increasing intestinal and gland activity
- Relaxing the muscles in the gastrointestinal tract

This system promotes calm and allows the body to perform self-healing and maintenance tasks that are deprioritized during stressful situations.

Doesn't that sound better? The purpose of this book is to give you the tools you need to spend plenty of time each day in parasympathetic mode. When you're in parasympathetic mode, you'll sleep better, have more balanced moods, enjoy flawless digestion, and experience relatively normal periods. Your weight will be regulated without much effort and your libido might even come back. You'll be released from the prison of **the Overs** and you'll start feeling better than you have in years.

I invite you to take a step back from the stressors of modern life and *think like the powerful women of your ancestral line*. Think of your great-great-great grandmother:

- Where did she live?
- What was her daily life like?
- What did she eat?
- How did she move her body?
- What did she spend her day doing?

## The Wisdom of Your Great-Great-Great Grandmother

Your ancestor's life likely looked much different from yours. Of course, it would be impossible to replicate ancestral life, and we wouldn't really want to. Hunger, disease, lack of indoor plumbing—no thank you! I'm glad to be a modern woman, and I'm thankful for the blessings that make my life easier. But although our lives may be *easier*, our ancestors' lives were *simpler*.

It's likely that your great-great-great grandmother woke easily around dawn and started preparing food for her family. She worked her body hard, but not in the gym. She walked regularly throughout the day, often outside. She lifted heavy things like children and tools. She ate regular meals. She knew that the labor of her hands depended on her internal and external strength. She drank water when she was thirsty.

Her body had to naturally adapt to the gentle stressors of heat and cold. She focused on her home, knowing that those who dwelled there would thrive under her care. She was productive with purpose throughout the day, and she slipped into bed at the end of the day, ready for a deep night's sleep.

This is the ideal, of course. Situations change. But the constants are similar—food, sun, sleep, and physical work. We'll dive deeper into these concepts throughout this book. I'll show you how you can channel Granny to navigate the confusing perimenopause journey and thrive throughout these years.

In the following chapters, you will learn practical steps to combat **the Overs** and finally get yourself out of fight-or-flight mode. You will receive action items that you can start using today to dial in your nutrition, exercise, and stress management. You'll get specific recommendations for food-based supplements, and I'll even give you a full 14-day meal plan to help you incorporate everything I'm teaching you. You probably never knew your great-great-great grandmother, but you'll learn plenty from her example over the following chapters.

# DEFINING TERMS:
## Your Hormones

## Hormones 101: The Hormone Family

Hormones are simply chemical messengers. They relay signals throughout the body. To understand hormones, think of them as members of a close-knit family, each with their unique roles and responsibilities. When everyone does their part, the household runs smoothly and harmoniously. For example:

- **Estrogen** is like the nurturing mother, ensuring everyone is well-fed and healthy.
- **Progesterone** is the calming father, keeping the household peaceful and ensuring everyone gets a good night's sleep.
- **Testosterone** is the energetic teenager, full of vim and vigor, always ready for action.
- **DHEA** is the supportive aunt, helping out wherever needed and filling in the gaps.
- **Pregnenolone** is the wise grandparent, providing wisdom and support for everyone's well-being.
- **Cortisol** is the diligent older sibling, managing stress and ensuring everything stays on track.
- **Adrenaline** is the quick-to-act uncle, ready to jump in during emergencies.

## How Stress Affects the Hormonal Family

Imagine that stress enters the household like an uninvited guest, causing chaos. The diligent older sibling, **Cortisol**, has to work overtime to manage the disruption. This extra workload means Cortisol can't perform her normal duties effectively, and she starts asking others for help:

- The nurturing mother, **Estrogen**, becomes distracted, affecting the family's overall health.
- The calming father, **Progesterone**, gets overwhelmed, leading to tension and sleepless nights.

- The energetic teenager, **Testosterone**, loses their vigor, feeling more tired and less motivated.
- The supportive aunt, **DHEA**, is stretched thin, unable to support everyone as before.
- The wise grandparent, **Pregnenolone**, becomes frazzled and struggles to provide the usual wisdom and support.
- The quick-to-act uncle, **Adrenaline**, is constantly on edge, ready to rush into every minor issue.

# Importance of Restoring Balance

Removing the source of stress and restoring harmony in the household is crucial. Without balance, everyone suffers, and the family's smooth functioning is disrupted. On the other hand, achieving hormonal balance helps you feel more energized, improves your mood, maintains your health, and ensures that all bodily functions proceed as they should.

Managing stress and focusing on overall well-being can help you restore this vital balance and enjoy a harmonious and healthy life.

While I prefer running the DUTCH for an optimal look at women's hormones, you can also ask your doctor to run a blood panel. Find the optimal blood ranges below.

# Estrogen

**Role in the body:**

- Regulates menstrual cycles and supports reproductive health
- Maintains bone density and skin health
- Influences mood and cognitive function

**Optimal blood lab range:**

- Follicular phase: 30–120 pg/mL
- Mid-cycle peak (ovulation): 130–400 pg/mL
- Luteal phase (post-ovulation): 70–250 pg/mL

# Progesterone

**Role in the body:**

- Balances the effects of estrogen and regulates menstrual cycles
- Supports pregnancy and embryo implantation
- Promotes calm and supports sleep

**Optimal blood lab range:**

- Follicular phase and post-menopause: 0.1–0.7 ng/mL
- Luteal phase (mid): 2–25 ng/mL

# Testosterone

**Role in the body:**

- Enhances libido and sexual function
- Supports muscle mass and strength
- Contributes to energy levels and mood stability

**Optimal blood lab range for total testosterone:**

- 15–70 ng/dL

# DHEA (Dehydroepiandrosterone)

**Role in the body:**

- Precursor to sex hormones like estrogen and testosterone
- Helps combat stress and fatigue
- Supports immune function and energy levels

**Optimal blood lab range:**

- 30–280 µg/dL

# Pregnenolone

**Role in the body:**

- Precursor to various hormones, including progesterone, estrogen, and cortisol
- Supports cognitive function and mood regulation
- Helps manage stress and inflammation

**Optimal blood lab range:**

- 22–237 ng/dL

# Cortisol

**Role in the body:**

- Regulates stress response and energy levels
- Controls blood sugar levels and metabolism
- Reduces inflammation

**Optimal blood lab range:**

- Morning (8 a.m.): 6–23 µg/dL
- Afternoon (4 p.m.): 3–15 µg/dL

# Adrenaline (Epinephrine)

**Role in the body:**

- Increases heart rate and blood flow during periods of high stress ("fight-or-flight" response)
- Boosts energy availability by breaking down glycogen
- Enhances physical performance during emergencies

**Optimal blood lab range:**

- Plasma adrenaline levels can vary, but typical resting levels are <50 pg/mL

# Banishing Over-Dieting – The New Guidelines for Proper Perimenopausal Nourishment

As CHILDREN OF the 1980s, many of us grew up around SnackWell's cookies, the Cabbage Soup Diet, and Weight Watchers. We watched our mothers religiously jump around to their workouts on VHS tapes. We were taught that fat was bad for us and that too many calories would make us chubby. Many of us restricted food from a young age, depriving ourselves of protein and increasing our chances of eventual malnourishment.

Now that we're in our thirties, forties, and fifties, we find it hard to let go of the dietary dogma that has been ingrained into our brains since we were dancing to Michael Jackson in neon T-shirts. In this chapter, we will explore why that very same low-calorie dietary dogma and the **Over-dieting** that results are contributing factors to many perimenopausal symptoms.

## *Gina*

Gina is a hustler. She rises before dawn, slips into her Lululemon, and meets a group of girlfriends to lead them through a workout almost every morning. These women have been dear friends for a long time, and their pre-sunrise sweat sessions are almost like therapy. They have supported each other through divorces and death, babies and grandbabies, joys and sorrows. The group relishes the smell of damp grass, and each woman feels her heart swell as the first rays of sunshine peek out from the distant hills. Therapy, indeed.

Gina loves taking care of others. She has raised three amazing young adults almost single-handedly. She's a teacher by trade, and thanks to her energy and warmth, she's beloved by students and colleagues alike.

Gina reflects my typical client. She is a high performer and a Type A achiever. She embodies the quote, "If you want something done, ask a busy person." Gina and I started working together years ago during the group coaching classes I run quarterly. While Gina looked amazing and felt pretty good, she had no idea that she was shortchanging herself of protein.

"Realizing that I should be eating nearly double the daily intake that I was blew my mind... IN A GOOD WAY!!!! I learned that eating more protein can not only boost weight loss but also enhance body composition! Also, as a woman in my fifties (athletic as I am), I found that my weight was creeping up. So, when I jumped into this reset, I was satisfied AND lost a few additional pounds at the same time."

Gina and I became each other's biggest fans, and she now helps me support other women as they learn to nourish themselves in perimenopause. For nearly every woman I work with, that includes eating more protein.

## The Importance of Protein

The word "protein" comes from the Greek word *proteus,* which means *of primary importance*. And this couldn't be more true!

Protein, fat, and carbohydrates are called **macronutrients**. These are the nutrients our bodies use in the largest amounts. Macronutrients are the basic units of food that our bodies need for energy and to maintain our bodies' structure and systems. Protein is arguably the most important macronutrient. Unfortunately, it's also the macronutrient that women tend to undereat regularly.

Dietary protein can be used as an energy source, but it's not very efficient in this role. Instead, our body uses dietary protein to repair and rebuild itself. Proteins are made up of chemical "building blocks" called amino acids, which our bodies use not only to build and repair muscles and bones but also to make hormones and enzymes. In perimenopause, it becomes even more important for women to consume enough protein to build and repair muscles and bones. It's also crucial to get enough protein to make healthy hormones like adrenaline, thyroid hormone, and melatonin.

## Cortisol, Insulin, and Stress

In midlife, we begin to feel the effects of t**he Overs**. One of the biggest issues with the Overs is that they are **catabolic**. "Catabolic" refers to the body's process of breaking things down. Remember cortisol? Cortisol is an extremely catabolic hormone. When stress levels are high, cortisol production can be constant. And when cortisol is regularly present in the bloodstream, muscle cells aren't able to absorb sugar and turn it into energy. Instead, cortisol starts to break down muscles to scavenge the little bits of energy stored there. The process of breaking down muscle protein to produce glucose (sugar) is called **gluconeogenesis**.

This is a one-two punch to the body because the process of pulling glucose into the bloodstream can also lead to **insulin resistance**, which happens when the bloodstream routinely carries excessive levels of sugar. **Insulin** is a hormone released from the pancreas that functions like a key. This key usually unlocks the cell, shuttling normal amounts of glucose inside the cell to be used for energy. However, when glucose levels are constantly elevated due to gluconeogenesis, insulin stops working as well. It can't effectively get glucose into the cells anymore, and the body starts diverting that glucose into your fat cells instead.

## An Insulin Analogy

Think of insulin as policemen and glucose as rioters. During a riot, the policemen are overrun by lawlessness and can no longer do their job effectively due to the large numbers of rioters. The jails (your cells) get quickly overrun by rioters (glucose). The body then has to shuttle the overflow of lawless people into a holding pen (your fat cells). The holding pen swells. The actual jail cells become crowded and ineffective. In the body, this looks like depleted energy and increased fat stores. This exact scenario—low energy and high fat stores—is the reality for so many perimenopausal women.

Stress is to blame.

But there's good news! We can mitigate much of this stress with a proper perimenopausal diet. And a proper perimenopausal diet starts with protein. Gina felt better equipped to handle the stressors of her day just by adding more protein to her meals. And her body responded in kind. It dropped a few pounds and began to change its composition. She felt more womanly again—her waist became more defined, and her curves became more apparent.

## Julie

Like Gina, Julie is a client who has done multiple month-long programs with me. She came into my program with intense sugar cravings, usually reaching a peak around 4 p.m. each day. I immediately recommended she get at least thirty grams of high-quality protein with each meal, and she dutifully added more meat to her day. Within a few weeks, she reported,

> *"When I get the right amount of protein, I do not have any cravings for other snacks. That has been a game changer for me."*

What would it look like…

- …if you didn't have any cravings for sugar?
- …if you didn't have to exercise major self-control to skip the chips and salsa every afternoon at 4 p.m.?
- …if you could set out a few cookies for your kids and not feel like you had to hide in the pantry, stuffing cookie after cookie into your mouth?

The simple act of adding more protein to your meals can help you do just that.

## *Stacy*

Stacy is a busy mom of two beautiful girls. One of her daughters is a college freshman, and the other recently got married and had a gorgeous baby girl named Georgia, making Stacy one of the youngest and cutest grandmothers I know. Like many of us, after Stacy's life got busy, she often found herself reaching for comfort foods to deal with the stress of her day-to-day activities. She craved sugar and foods that she knew were not good for her. She knew that these foods made her less energetic and more moody.

Stacy has done many of my programs and loves returning to the protein-centric meal plans of Easy Perimenopause. She knows when she's on a plan, she won't struggle with the sugar demon.

> *"Eating more protein fuels me and keeps me from craving all the SUGAR!! Now when I start looking for empty-calorie foods, I try to ask myself 'How much protein have you eaten today?' Then I try to head to the leftover meats or lunch meats and snack on those instead."*

Years of training herself to reach for protein first have helped her keep her figure fit and her energy high, so she can continue to love her family and her friends well.

## Protein, Cravings, and Weight Loss

I can tell you to eat more protein (*and I am telling you to eat more protein!*), but it's helpful for you to know *why* I'm encouraging you to do so. It's quite possible that you picked up this book because you're concerned about your recent perimenopausal weight gain. You're not alone. By 2026, nearly

401 million perimenopausal women in our country will face a heightened risk of menopausal obesity (1). This will be a double-whammy for so many of us as we're forced to deal with not only annoying menopausal symptoms but also the long-term metabolic issues associated with obesity.

Weight gain at this stage in life is often due to middle-aged women's lack of awareness about their own health. We tend to prioritize our families' well-being over our own. This neglect makes it difficult for many women to start any weight loss efforts and can worsen the issue of weight gain.

Before perimenopause, women generally have normal estrogen levels in their bodies at any given time. But as we transition through perimenopause and into menopause, those estrogen levels begin to decline. One estrogen's effects is inhibiting hunger signals. Naturally, when we don't feel as hungry, we don't eat as much. In perimenopause, declining estrogen means that our body is unable to regulate hunger hormones. Our intensified hunger signals cause us to eat more.

As we transition toward menopause, we also start to accumulate the dreaded "perimenopause belly." This is a hallmark of perimenopause for so many women who feel confused and frustrated by the fact that their diet and exercise routines are no longer working for them. Clothes don't fit, sex feels embarrassing, and confidence is affected as they try in vain to stuff that lower belly pooch into shapewear or clothes that are now too small. Newly lowered estrogen levels that occur during this time and increasing levels of androgenic hormones like testosterone also lead to fat redistribution (2). Padding that was previously and preferably in our butt and thighs makes its way to our lower belly.

When we feel bad about ourselves, we often make decisions that make us feel better in the moment. Lifestyle-related factors that increase perimenopausal weight gain include eating too much food, not eating enough fiber, skipping meals and then eating large meals, irregular sleep, and too much alcohol.

Skimping on protein can cause weight gain, but it can also cause a decline in muscle mass. In perimenopause, the metabolism starts to slow down, and women can no longer burn calories at the higher metabolic rate they enjoyed as younger women. Many women at this stage of life are also dealing with low thyroid function and hormonal disorders like PCOS that can be primary reasons for weight gain.

*Increasing dietary protein is a first-line defense in fighting perimenopausal weight gain.* Some studies suggest getting at least 25% of your daily calories from protein, but other studies raise that number to 30% or more (3). On a 2,000-calorie-a-day diet, that can mean getting up to 150 grams of protein. Don't be scared; you can start slowly.

I recommend that women start adding more protein to their diet by ensuring breakfast, lunch, and dinner all include at least thirty grams of protein (for guidance, refer to the 14-day suggested meal plan toward the end of this book). If you are getting that much protein, you'll feel so nourished and satisfied that you won't be craving the chips, ice cream, and wine like you used to.

Protein is key to shutting off cravings. In fact, one study showed that when 40-year-olds with an average body mass index (BMI) of 34 ate a diet containing 28% protein, food cravings were significantly reduced by week four of the diet (4). A meta-analysis of 68 studies showed that a high-protein diet decreased hunger and desire to eat while increasing feelings of fullness and satiety. It also revealed that getting plenty of protein decreased ghrelin, the hormone associated with hunger.

Enough protein also increases glucagon-like peptide-1 (GLP-1). You know what else mimics GLP-1? Semaglutide, the shiny new shot your cousin and best friend are using to lose lots of weight. If you eat plenty of protein in combination with a moderate-calorie, high-nourishment diet, you won't need to spend $1,000 a month on a potentially dangerous weight loss shot (5, 6). I call that a win!

## Protein and Sleep

Another benefit of protein is that it can help perimenopausal women sleep more deeply. Later in this book, we'll be taking a whole chapter to cover sleep. But for now, you should know that getting between 100 to 150 grams of animal protein a day can help stabilize your blood sugar and increase sleep-inducing hormones like tryptophan.

One well-designed study pitted a diet containing 10% protein against a 30% protein diet (7). Not only did the researchers find that the group eating 30% protein had more lean muscle mass by the end of the 90-day study, but they also found that every measure of sleep quality improved in the high protein group. The group eating 30% of their diet as protein fell asleep faster, experienced better oxygen delivery to tissues, and even snored less than the control group.

## Protein and Brain Health

Protein has a beautifully beneficial effect on another frustrating casualty of perimenopause—brain health. Every day, I talk to women who complain of depression, anxiety, anger, and brain fog. These women are worried about the current state of their brains, and they're also fearful that the coming years will bring neurodegeneration and diseases like Alzheimer's or Parkinson's. Perimenopause is the perfect time to start fighting back against declining brain health.

A high-protein diet can actually initiate positive short- and long-term changes in the neurons of the brain (8) by increasing the brain's creation of energy as measured by adenosine triphosphate (ATP) (9). ATP is often called the "energy currency" of the cell because it provides energy that's easy for cells to access. And a brain with plenty of energy is a focused, well-functioning brain. Eating a protein-rich diet ensures that you're getting a steady supply of **amino acids**—the building blocks of dietary protein—to the body and the brain.

The amino acids tyrosine and phenylalanine are necessary to begin the brain's production of **dopamine**, a neurotransmitter associated with feelings of pleasure and contentment. When it's low, we tend to feel depressed, anxious, and even angry. I routinely test my clients' dopamine levels and usually these levels are quite low. One of the first interventions I'll use for low dopamine is *more dietary protein*.

Tryptophan is another amino acid we get from protein-rich foods. Tryptophan converts to 5-hydroxytryptophan (5-HTP) in the body, which then converts to serotonin. Serotonin is the brain neurotransmitter that helps us feel joyful. If you're on a traditional antidepressant, that medication is working in the brain to recycle what little serotonin you may be making.

Twenty percent of women over forty are currently on an antidepressant (10); meanwhile, millions of other perimenopausal women are suffering from anxiety and depression in silence or are attempting to self-medicate through supplements, alcohol, or even street drugs. Recent research shows that the average American woman is eating about 69 grams of protein each day (11). It's no surprise that we're suffering from mood disorders and poor brain health when we're only getting (at best) 69% of the protein our bodies are crying out for. *Sixty-nine percent is a "D" grade in school.* And we're overachievers around here, right? We all want that "A" grade in Protein Class. So, work on getting at least 100 grams of protein each day.

## Potassium: The Other Perimenopausal "P"

Protein is primary, yes. But let's talk about our other perimenopausal "P" word—**potassium**, a crucial electrolyte and dietary mineral that's needed for a variety of functions throughout the body. It's especially important for perimenopausal women because it contributes to bone density, muscle relaxation, quality sleep, and fluid balance. Without sufficient potassium, we can become bloated, puffy, and irritable. We can also become quite hungry!

My clients know this to be true. For instance, Kate had trouble sleeping through the night. Like many of my clients, when she first got in bed, she could fall asleep just fine. But she woke up every night around 1 a.m. and had trouble getting back to sleep. We started her on electrolytes and within a few weeks, Kate reported,

> *"I'm sleeping so much better since I added the potassium electrolytes."*

Rachel also battled sleep issues for years. She tossed and turned for hours each night, agonizing over the lack of sleep and wondering how she was going to show up with energy and love to serve the students at the school she's taught at for years. I recommended immediate electrolyte intervention via the Adrenal Cocktail. Three weeks after our first meeting, Rachel told me,

> *"The adrenal cocktail helps relax and calm my body and prepare it for sleep."*

*(P.S. The recipe for this potassium-rich Adrenal Cocktail can be found in a later chapter!)*

I love the positive effects of potassium so much that I also recommend it to everyone around me. My dear friend Mayra told me that her son, Jason, suffered from muscle cramps that would regularly take him out of his varsity football games. Jason is a star receiver and the team needed his speed and strength to win. I suggested that Mayra regularly give Jason potassium-rich electrolytes, and his muscle cramps immediately got better.

Intrigued, Mayra started taking the electrolytes too. At 46, she noticed she was feeling more tired each afternoon. Her history of running marathons and her current early-morning workout schedule were catching up with her, and she felt like she needed to take a nap every afternoon. Within a few days of adding potassium-rich electrolytes to her water bottle, she was amazed to tell me,

> *"I've had so much energy in the afternoons! Instead of taking a nap, I'm scrubbing baseboards and washing windows."*

Mayra continues to drink her electrolyte powder to this day.

The recommended daily intake of potassium has changed in the past five years. Before 2019, government officials recommended that adults consume 4,700 mg per day. But then the guidelines were updated to recommend far less potassium—only 2,600 mg per day for adult females. Why?

> *"[The government] established AIs for all ages based on the highest median potassium intakes in healthy children and adults and on estimates of potassium intakes from breast milk and complementary foods in infants" (11).*

While the median potassium intake for relatively healthy people may be only 2,600 mg per day, that number is certainly not optimal.

# Marty Kendall and the Optimal Nutrition Intake

How do we know that 2,600 mg a day of potassium is not optimal? Through the work of Marty Kendall, a brilliant engineer and researcher who sought to help his wife, Monica, use nutrition to better control her Type 1 diabetes. After successfully helping Monica manage her disease and lose weight, he began helping others optimize their nutrition by consuming optimal levels of both macronutrients and micronutrients as well as working on blood sugar balance.

Marty has collected nutrition data from thousands of individuals through his work. With plenty of evidence, he developed a framework that he calls the **optimal nutritional intake** (ONI). The ONI looks quite different from government recommendations, like the Recommended Daily Allowance (RDA). The RDA is the average amount of a vitamin or mineral a person needs to consume daily to meet their nutrient requirements; theoretically, it is the average intake that is sufficient to meet the nutrient requirements of 97 to 98 percent of "healthy" people. (Ask yourself: how many truly "healthy" people do you know? Are *you* healthy?)

However, research shows that the RDA is set far too low for most nutrients and a small proportion of the U.S. population consumes a nutritionally adequate diet (12). The RDA doesn't consider age, location, activity levels, chronic health conditions, or the way nutrients interact with each other. As such, the RDA does not reflect optimal levels. Marty's ONI paints a much more comprehensive picture of what a person needs to feel their best. Instead of focusing on consuming enough micronutrients to prevent disease, like the RDA, Marty's daily nutrient suggestions aim to help people *thrive*.

Potassium is a huge player in helping people thrive, especially women in perimenopause. This is due to the fact that potassium can greatly increase feelings of satiety or fullness. "If you get foods that naturally contain more potassium per calorie, you can eat less, and it's definitely a significant nutrient in the satiety factors," says Marty. His comprehensive analysis of tens of thousands of people suggests that those who eat more higher potassium foods may eat up to 40% fewer calories.

Women who take in an average of 1,800 mg of potassium per day can easily eat almost 2,100 calories. But Marty's data shows that consuming potassium-rich foods to reach the ONI of 4,200 mg of potassium and 2,000 calories can translate to eating almost 40% fewer calories.

This is fascinating work! We women work doggedly to deprive ourselves of calories in a futile effort to lose weight. Still hungry, we force ourselves, meal after meal, to stop eating with the hope that we'll wake up a little thinner the next morning. But we have it wrong. Women should not be trying to *take away*. We should be trying to *add*. Contributing both protein and minerals like potassium to functionally starving bodies is the first step toward achieving true metabolic health.

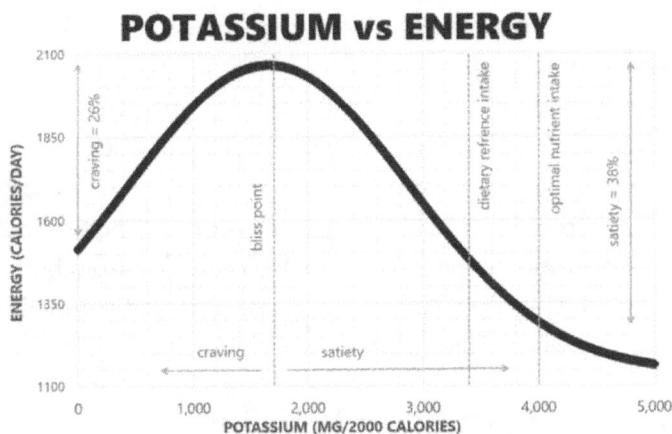

## POTASSIUM vs ENERGY

Table 1: At the ONI level of 4,200 mg of dietary potassium, eating fewer calories becomes effortless. Reprinted with permission from Marty Kendall.

## Further Research

The research is clear on this subject. Three different studies have shown that higher consumption of potassium correlated with a lower prevalence of obesity (13, 14, 15). In the Dallas Heart Study, a higher intake of potassium was associated with lower levels of body fat (16). A study from *Obesity* found correlations between higher potassium intake, smaller waist size, and a lower body mass index (BMI) (17).

# How to Get More Potassium

Foods high in potassium include bananas, of course. This is the food that most people think of when they hear the word "potassium." However, three ounces of tuna actually contains more potassium (118 mg) than one medium banana (105 mg). One small white potato has 128 mg of potassium, one cup of low-fat yogurt has 143 mg, and one medium sweet potato contains 105 mg.

Animal products are especially rich in potassium. Six ounces of 95% fat free ground beef has 588 mg of potassium. Six ounces of turkey has 408 mg. And 6 ounces of chicken has 379 mg. Meat contains as much (or more) potassium as many fruits and vegetables, so don't shy away from beef, especially if you're trying to stay out of fight-or-flight mode and manage cravings.

# What About Plant Protein?

My friend Theresa is an ethical vegetarian. She has a "rescue cow" named Baxter and a "rescue goat" named Bart. Her morals prevent her from eating animals. She is healthy and fit and pays close attention to her diet, getting plenty of protein from eggs and dairy products and plant sources.

If you are ethically plant-based like Theresa, I understand the commitment to doing what you think is right. However, I can say from clinical experience that most plant-based women are not getting enough protein, and many of them are getting too many refined and processed carbohydrates. It's very hard for most women to get over 100 grams of plant-based protein!

As a women's hormone expert, I prefer that my hormon-ally-imbalanced women regularly eat thoughtfully raised animal products. Animal protein is an ancestral food that is extremely beneficial for women. Why?

Animal protein is better at helping women attain and maintain lean muscle mass (18).

Animal protein is easier to digest than plant protein, which means we absorb more of it. Plant-based proteins are also lower in essential and nonessential amino acids (19). The work of Dr. Georgia Ede, a Harvard-trained psychiatrist specializing in nutritional and metabolic psychiatry, strongly advocates for meat consumption among women due to its comprehensive nutritional benefits. She emphasizes that meat provides essential nutrients that are either absent or less bioavailable in plant-based foods.

Dr. Ede argues that these nutrients are difficult to obtain in adequate amounts from plant-based diets alone, and their deficiencies can adversely affect physical and mental health. She notes that meat is the only food that contains every nutrient we need in its proper form and is also the safest food for our blood sugar and insulin levels.

I was lucky enough to have Dr. Ede as my teacher for three months, and I learned so many things from her! One thing I learned from my time with Dr. Ede is that meat truly is a superfood. Consider this infographic:

Micronutrient Availability in Plant and Animal Foods

| | |
|---|---|
| Vitamin A | 12 to 24 times more bioavailable in animal foods |
| Vitamins B1, B2, B3, B6, B7 | Easier to find in animal foods |
| Vitamin B9 (Folate) | Insoluble matrix in some plant foods hinders bioavailability |
| Vitamin B12 | Not found in plant foods |
| Vitamin C | Easier to find in plant foods |
| Vitamin D | D3 from animal foods easier to use/store than D2 from fungi and yeast |
| Vitamin E | Easier to find in plant foods |
| Vitamin K1 | Easier to find in plant foods |
| Vitamin K2 | Not found in plant foods (except in a few fermented foods, e.g. natto) |
| Iron | Bioavailability of heme iron (15–35%) is greater than non-heme iron (2–20%). Eggs, dairy, and many plants contain compounds that interfere with iron absorption |
| Calcium | Some plants contain compounds that interfere with calcium absorption |
| Iodine | Many plants contain compounds that interfere with iodine utilization |
| Zinc | Many plants contain compounds that interfere with zinc absorption |
| EPA and DHA | Not found in plant foods. Plant foods contain ALA, which must be converted to EPA and DHA. Conversion of ALA to EPA is low: 8% in men and up to 21% in women. Conversion of ALA to DHA is very low: 0-4% in men and 9% in women |

Table 2: Bioavailability of nutrients in animal products and plant products. Reprinted with permission from Dr. Georgia Ede.

At the end of the day, your decision whether or not to eat meat is highly personal. But after working with thousands of perimenopausal women, I can say that the majority of women thrive on an animal protein-inclusive diet.

## Shutting Down Cravings

Animal protein can be very effective at shutting down intense sugar cravings. My client, Lana, spent a month consciously increasing her protein intake to well over 100 grams a day. She had previously been struggling with perimenopausal weight gain and sugar cravings. Lana wanted to model healthy eating habits for her daughter and was frustrated that she felt so bad. So, we started her on the Easy Perimenopause plan. Within a month, she reported back:

*"I've lost eight pounds, sleep well, my clothes are way more comfy... my cravings are much less, and I feel satisfied."*

Michelle fared similarly. As she worked to increase her protein intake over the course of a month, she reported, "My cravings and impulsive eating stopped." Thanks to Marty Kendall, we know that this shutdown of cravings isn't necessarily due to the satiation factor of animal protein alone. It's also because animal protein is high in minerals like potassium, which helps shut down cravings.

What would it mean for you if you stopped struggling with cravings? Would you be able to let go of the shame of hiding your secret pantry binges from your kids and husband? Would you feel the freedom that comes with finishing a meal and being completely satisfied, instead of mentally planning how you will execute your sugar binge alone in the pantry after your family has gone to bed? Will you feel confident passing by the candy jar at work without a second thought, instead of rationing out how many times a day you can sneak a piece without someone seeing you?

Freedom from cravings means freedom from the prison of food and dieting. Eating to fuel your body instead of eating compulsively or for entertainment can help you experience a safety and contentment that you likely have not known before, especially if you've been immersed in diet culture for years or decades.

It's simple: get 100+ grams of animal protein every single day and aim to get between 4,000 and 6,000 mg of potassium each day. Use a free smartphone app like Cronometer to track your food for a few days—not out of a desire to rigidly track calories, but from the gamified perspective of giving yourself a gold star every time you eat enough protein and potassium. Start there and watch your cravings fade away.

When I really dialed in my protein and made sure to eat at least 30–35 grams with each meal, my sugar cravings subsided dramatically. I felt fuller for a longer time and no longer had that gnawing hunger in my stomach between meals. I felt full and satisfied and thought about food less often than when I was eating less protein. But I was still struggling with afternoon fatigue.

It wasn't until I learned about potassium and started getting 4,000–5,000 mg of potassium a day that my energy skyrocketed. I no longer felt like taking afternoon naps. My workouts got stronger, my recovery time decreased, and I felt the genuine desire to be active more often throughout the day. Because I mistreated my adrenal glands for so many years, my body craves a lot of salt. I knew sodium was good for me, but potassium was the missing piece. Sodium by itself made me feel bloated and caused me to retain water. When I focused on getting more potassium-rich foods into my diet, I lost my puffy water weight and no longer felt bloated.

I started making Potassium Broth once a week and drinking two cups each afternoon (with added salt, naturally!). This got me to 2,000 mg of potassium each day. I also focused on eating plenty of potatoes, bananas, avocados, and meat. This helped round out my goal of 4,000–5,000 mg of potassium daily. I used Cronometer to track this—get the link at **www.jenniferwoodwardnutrition.com/resources**.

# Potassium Recipes

These are the potassium-rich recipes that helped me dial in my energy and lose the water weight. Start with one cup of Potassium Broth each afternoon. Work up to two cups daily. After a few weeks, if you're still craving potassium, add in the Potassium Smoothie for an after-dinner snack.

The Potassium Broth is an easy addition to the recommended meal plan I have for you at the end of this book. It is virtually calorie-free and can be sipped on in the afternoon. If you're adding in the Potassium Smoothie, simply omit the suggested dessert and substitute the Potassium Smoothie for any day of the plan.

## Potassium Broth

Potassium broth is a nourishing and mineral-rich broth packed with essential nutrients. Here's a simple recipe with approximately 1,000 mg of potassium per serving:

**Ingredients:**

- 4 large potatoes, with skins (approximately 2,000 mg of potassium)
- 2 large carrots (approximately 100 mg of potassium)
- 2 stalks celery (approximately 200 mg of potassium)
- 1 large onion
- 1 cup chopped spinach (approximately 250 mg of potassium)
- 2 cloves garlic
- 1 teaspoon sea salt
- 1 teaspoon black pepper
- 8 cups water

**Instructions:**

- Wash all vegetables thoroughly. Ensure the potato skins remain on, as they are rich in potassium.
- Cut potatoes into quarters, slice carrots and celery, and chop the onion into large pieces.
- Mince garlic cloves.
- In a large pot, add all the prepared vegetables, garlic, and spinach.
- Pour in 8 cups of water and stir to combine.
- Add sea salt and black pepper for flavor.
- Bring the mixture to a boil over high heat.
- Once boiling, reduce heat to a simmer.
- Cover the pot and allow it to simmer for about one hour. This helps extract the nutrients from the vegetables into the broth.
- After simmering, remove from heat.
- Strain the broth through a fine mesh strainer or cheesecloth into another pot or large bowl, removing all solids.

Store any leftover broth in an airtight container in the refrigerator for up to three days or freeze for later use.

## Potassium Smoothie

This smoothie contains approximately 1,000 mg of potassium:

**Ingredients:**

- 1 medium avocado, peeled (approximately 480 mg of potassium)
- 1 large banana, peeled (approximately 400 mg of potassium)
- 1 cup coconut water (approximately 600 mg of potassium)
- 1/2 cup spinach (optional, approximately 80 mg of potassium)
- 1 tablespoon chia seeds (optional for added nutrients)
- 1 cup ice
- 1 teaspoon honey or liquid stevia to taste (optional for sweetness)

**Instructions:**
Mix all ingredients in a high-powered blender and serve.

# Nutrition Action Items

- Aim to eat at least 100 grams of high-quality animal protein per day. Use the recipes and meal plans suggested in this book to help you meet your daily protein goal. If you really want that gold star, aim for one gram of protein per pound of desired body weight. For instance, if a normal weight for your height and body type is 145 pounds, try to eat 145 grams of protein each day.
- Start your day with at least 30 grams of protein. Eat breakfast within 30 minutes of waking up.

- Add in the **Potassium Broth** each afternoon and consider adding the **Potassium Smoothie** as your after-dinner snack.
- Use a food tracking app like Cronometer to ensure you get at least 4,700 mg of potassium each day.

## CHAPTER 3:

# Over-Tired – How To Start Sleeping Better Tonight

WHEN I WAS a teenager struggling with the stress of playing year-round sports, working a job, and maintaining my 4.0+ GPA, my father used to tell me, *"Nobody ever died from lack of sleep."* I took my father's advice to heart. In college, I would stay up late to study (or party). In my early motherhood years, I would cling to the idea that even though I was up every hour with crying babies, I wouldn't die from the lack of sleep. But that lack of sleep gets old, fast. And as I got older, I realized that there's a good reason why sleep deprivation is used as a form of torture. Women in perimenopause are particularly vulnerable to this torture.

## The Research on Sleep

A study by the American Academy of Sleep Medicine echoed my suspicion–it's not just me. Turns out, women are drowning in this haze of exhaustion at a rate that overshadows men: around 32% of us toss and turn through the night compared to their 21%. The majority of women (81%) report that sleepiness affects their daily activities (1).

Sleep disturbances are one of the top symptoms my clients report when we start working together. After age forty, most women suffer from the frustrations of not being able to fall asleep, not being able to stay asleep, or both.

This makes sense. When we don't prioritize sleep, we have a hard time sleeping well. Sleep isn't a switch that we can turn on and off. We have to practice the habits that lead to a good night's sleep. And ideally, we should be doing so all day long.

Our modern lifestyles conspire against us. Every incoming stimulus throughout the day—caffeine, inadequate nutrition, rushing everywhere, exercising, and blue light from phone and television screens—tells our brain that it's daytime. When it is daytime, the brain needs to be active. The body needs to be active. Hormones like cortisol and adrenaline are constantly excreted to meet these demands. But when these hormones are elevated at night, the resulting imbalance is referred to as an *altered diurnal cortisol pattern*.

## Understanding Cortisol

In healthy women, cortisol secretion follows a "diurnal" pattern in which levels are highest upon waking, increase significantly during the morning, and steadily decrease from the peak throughout the rest of the day, reaching their lowest levels in the middle of the night. Cortisol patterns are described as "diurnal" because cortisol secretion should be happening during the day. When something happens at night, it is referred to as "nocturnal" (2). The natural ebb and flow of daytime and nighttime hormone secretion is called our **circadian rhythm** (derived from the Latin *circa* (about) and *dies* (day)).

The constant state of fight-or-flight experienced by many perimenopausal women means daytime stressors push cortisol secretion into the evening hours and prevent us from getting to sleep. Cortisol can increase attentiveness and wakefulness. It can also stimulate our muscle cells and liver to release glucose, temporarily raising and then dropping blood sugar levels. All of these effects of cortisol tell our bodies that it is time to be awake, not to sleep.

Our daytime stressors become our waking nightmares, as lack of sleep conspires to make us exhausted, depressed, anxious, irritable, and hungry. This is a further frustration for the perimenopausal female, as more than sleep is affected when our diurnal cortisol pattern is out of whack. Cortisol itself acts to synchronize the "clocks" in the liver, muscle, fat tissue, pancreas, and gut (3).

A balanced nervous system is a prerequisite for consistently restful sleep. *In this book, reducing high cortisol levels is the primary way we'll work on your sleep.*

If we want to get really nerdy, we can talk about the **suprachiasmatic nucleus** of the brain. This is a small group of neurons in the hypothalamus that controls the body's circadian rhythm, including sleep. It also contains a large quantity of estrogen receptors (4). So, when estrogen levels fluctuate wildly, as they do in perimenopause, it becomes harder for our bodies to maintain normal sleep schedules and circadian rhythms. This is why it's especially important for women over the age of 40 to practice healthy sleep hygiene.

## Practical Sleep Strategies

Simply establishing a regular sleep schedule can be the first step toward getting better sleep. In our twenties, we could wake up at 4:30 a.m. on the weekdays and sleep until 10 a.m. on the weekends. But it's rare for a perimenopausal woman to be able to "sleep in," especially if she's getting up early on weekdays.

I hope you're already reconsidering that early wake time—remember, at this point in life, your hormones would rather have sleep, not an early morning workout. Moderate and regular exercise during daytime hours after eating a good breakfast or lunch can enhance sleep. We'll talk about hormone-friendly exercise in Chapter 4. For now, consider setting your alarm for about 6 a.m. every morning, regardless of what day it is.

Years ago, after I had four children within a six year span, my sister-in-law Staci encouraged me to get each of my four babies on a "sleep schedule" as early as possible. This set both mama and the newborn up for success; we both established intrinsic rhythms of *eat, wake, play, sleep.* Perimenopausal women thrive on similar routines. Our hormones need rhythms and stability. Sleep is one of the first things to suffer when our rhythms are off.

## Morning Routine

A regular "wake time" is the first priority when pursuing a great night's sleep.

## Get Early Morning Sunlight

After getting up at a consistent time, **try to expose yourself to early morning sunlight as quickly as possible.** Full-spectrum light from the sun sets into motion a beautifully orchestrated circadian rhythm. Morning light tells your brain to begin the hormone cascade of creating serotonin (our happiness neurotransmitter) (4).

# Eat Protein Soon After Waking

This process is also dependent on tryptophan, an essential amino acid. In this context, "essential" means we can only get tryptophan through food; animal-based protein foods are very high in tryptophan (5). So, waking up, preparing yourself some eggs and turkey sausage, and sitting on your front porch to expose yourself to early morning sunlight while enjoying a quiet start to your day will actually help you sleep better at night!

# Eat Regular, Nourishing Meals

Another way to calm the stress response and sleep better later at night is to eat regular, nourishing meals during the day. The research clearly demonstrates this. In a study of 121 women, restricting calories increased total cortisol output. Interestingly (and unsurprisingly), even the act of monitoring calories increased stress perception (6). Additional studies corroborate this data in both cycling and postmenopausal women (7, 8).

Restricting calories is stressful and the body responds to this stress by releasing cortisol. To prevent the release of excess cortisol, stop dieting. Stop worrying about every calorie you put in your mouth. Just make sure to get at least 100 grams of high-quality protein every day. Don't skip breakfast, and don't drink coffee on an empty stomach. Without food in your stomach, the caffeine jolt from coffee can spike your cortisol, putting you into fight-or-flight mode first thing in the morning.

## Honor Your Sleepiness

Eating regular meals can help you keep your diurnal cortisol pattern stable, helping you to start feeling sleepy at normal times. You should ideally start feeling tired around 9 p.m. and be in bed and asleep by 10 p.m. There is some leeway here. Optimal sleep means something different for everyone—it's the amount of sleep you need to optimize your performance, brain power, mood, physical health, and quality of life (9).

Rest assured that skimping on your sleep will affect your nervous system negatively, too. I've had many clients who tell me that the wee hours of the morning are their "me time." After the kids go to bed, they just want to (or need to) clean, watch TV, check their emails, scroll through Instagram, or drink wine. This habit can destroy your circadian rhythm while robbing you of quality sleep.

## Get to Bed by 10

It might take some intentional retraining to get to bed before 10 p.m., but it can be done. It's one of the most important things you can do for hormonal balance. Sleep trumps everything—diet, exercise, and even nervous system rebalancing. When you're working on a great night's sleep throughout the day, slumber becomes easy and satisfying. Your great-great-great grandmother didn't have to deal with the blue light emanating from nighttime screens. She had to conserve her candles and gas lamps. When the sun went down, activity slowed down. Bedtime was a welcome respite from the hard work of the day. We want to emulate those routines.

Hopefully, at this point, you're already starting to consider increasing your protein and calorie intake so that your nervous system can balance out enough to help you fall asleep easily. You're thinking about getting early morning sun. And you're not pushing heavy exercise on a coffee-fueled stomach. These are great things to do during the day. Let's talk about sleep-enhancing nighttime activities, too.

# Evening Routine

As evening approaches, try to turn off all screens by 9 p.m. so you have a good hour to devote to sleep hygiene.

# Take a Hot Bath

Start by taking a hot Epsom salt bath. Take a bath with water as hot as you can safely handle. Try to stay submerged for fifteen to twenty minutes. I like to lay a towel down on my bathroom floor and cover myself with another towel. I'll rest there for about ten minutes as my body cools down and I get back to equilibrium. This prepares me well for sleep. If you don't like baths or if you don't have a tub, buy an inexpensive foot bath and use it as directed. *(P.S. In Chapter 5, you're going to get my complete slumber-inducing bath time routine.)*

# Get Off Screens

After you've cooled down, continue your bedtime routine by putting on natural fiber pajamas and crawling into bed with a good book (or a magazine, if books aren't your jam). Stay away from the blue light that phones and TVs emanate.

This blue light tells your body that it's day, not night, and will send the wrong message to your brain.

## Sex and Stretching

If you're still too amped up to sleep, consider doing some gentle stretching or yoga. If you feel like it, grab your man and get physical; a recent study shows that sex with your partner reduces cortisol levels in women specifically (interestingly enough, however, this effect is blunted for women on birth control) (10). Stressed at bedtime? Instead of stewing on it, tell your husband that sex is good for your cortisol levels and watch him light up!

## Have a Snack

Oftentimes, a woman's cortisol levels are still high at bedtime because she has not had enough to eat during the day. If you've already tried everything else, one of the most effective ways to induce sleep is to eat something before bed. A healthy and balanced snack includes small amounts of protein, fat, and carbohydrates.

An example would be a tablespoon of nut butter on half an apple or banana, or one cup of baby carrots with two slices of turkey lunch meat. These balanced snacks lower cortisol levels, helping sleep to come more easily. Eat your snack and go to bed. If you struggle with night waking, leave some nuts and dried fruit by your bedside table.

If you wake up at night and cannot go back to sleep, eat a small handful of almonds and raisins or cashews and dates (any combination of fruit and dried nuts that you prefer), take a sip of water, use the restroom, and then get back into bed.

You should fall asleep easily as the cortisol response lowers. It's likely that you won't have to use this hack every night, or even for an extended period of time. As your nervous system rebalances in a few weeks and you start sleeping better, you won't need a snack in the middle of the night.

# Kick Alcohol to the Curb

I'm going to give it to you straight: alcohol also disrupts your sleep. Inherently, most women know this to be true. But the research backs it up. A two-year study with over 3,500 participants found that women who drank more than 21 units of alcohol a week had significantly higher cortisol levels than men who drank the equivalent amount of alcohol, and that even one drink a day raised cortisol levels (11). In this study, a "unit" is defined as 8 grams of ethanol. This is the equivalent of 4.2 oz of wine, 12 ounces of 5% alcohol by volume (ABV) beer, or 1.5 ounces of hard alcohol.

A standard bottle of wine contains six full servings. So, if every night, you drink half of a bottle of wine, you would be characterized as a *heavy drinker* according to this study. Until I quit drinking alcohol, I could drink most of a bottle of wine every night without even realizing it. I felt both refined and sassy for about an hour, and then I would spend hours and hours in bed, literally and metaphorically sweating my alcohol.

Another study echoed this finding: When women drink alcohol, they produce more cortisol than men (12). Women are more susceptible to the negative effects of alcohol on the nervous system. This is why when you and your husband have drinks at dinner, he can sleep like a baby and experience no existential crisis while you're sweating through your sheets and wide awake at 3 a.m., vowing you'll never drink again.

We don't want to raise cortisol at night. Alcohol raises cortisol.

## Alcohol Reduces REM Sleep

Another meta-analysis on women and alcohol showed that moderate intake of alcohol reduced the amount of time women spent in the restorative rapid eye movement (REM) part of their sleep cycle. Total sleep time also decreased, while the frequency of night wakings increased. The researchers found that men did not experience any differences in total sleep time, REM, or night wakings as a result of drinking alcohol (13). Women respond to alcohol differently than men. It affects our cortisol levels and our sleep differently. If you're truly passionate about getting a good night's sleep, consider giving up alcohol.

## Functional Lab Testing

Saliva or urine hormone testing can reveal a clear picture of stress hormone patterns over a twenty-four-hour period. These tests often reveal that my clients have elevated cortisol levels at night. They can see that their bodies are too stressed to sleep! Seeing this data in black and white makes it much easier to guide clients as they create effective bedtime routines tailored to their specific needs.

# I'm Getting My Best Sleep in Years

With these tips, you should be able to manage and mitigate nighttime cortisol levels which can help you sleep better than ever. I'm happy to say that in my forties, my sleep is deeper and more restful than it was in my twenties or thirties. I prioritize my sleep hygiene so noticeably that my dear friend Neddy bought me a porch mat that says, "Welcome! Please leave by 9."

I love sleeping through the night and waking up refreshed. While I didn't die from lack of sleep in the previous decades, I certainly felt like the walking dead for many years. But now, I routinely practice everything I've taught you in this chapter and I am a happy, well-rested mama. If you put these action steps into place, you too can be happy and well-rested within a few weeks.

# Rest/Sleep Action Items

- Wake up at the same time every morning if possible.
- Expose your eyes and body to early morning sunlight for at least 10 minutes each morning—sun, rain, or snow.
- Eat a balanced, protein-rich breakfast as soon as possible after waking. Eating calms the stress response. Don't drink coffee on an empty stomach. Have it with your breakfast instead.
- Eat three balanced, protein-rich meals every day.
- Consider breaking up with alcohol for good.
- Take a mineral-rich Epsom salt bath before bed.
- Get into bed by 10 p.m. each night.

- Have a snack before bed to prevent night waking. If woken in the middle of the night and unable to get back to sleep, have a quick balanced snack and go back to bed.

# Banishing Over-Exercise – The New Rules for Exercise in the Perimenopausal Years

On a cold Tuesday morning in 2013, my alarm clock went off at 4:45 a.m. I dragged myself out of my cozy bed. My comforter felt particularly soft that morning, and I was groggy after being abruptly woken from a dream. I glanced over at my sleeping husband, jealous that he was still peacefully snoring.

I got up every morning before the sun rose so that I could jog for at least forty-five minutes. My day started quickly, with four children needing breakfast before we began our homeschool activities. If I didn't get my run in early, it didn't happen. And I loved to check things off of my to-do list—workouts most of all. It gave me a deep satisfaction to have completed this healthy activity before most of the world even emerged from their bedrooms.

But I was *tired*. Every day around 2 p.m., I would hit a wall. It didn't matter that I'd had three or four cups of coffee throughout the morning. By the early afternoon, I was mentally and physically checked out. My limbs dragged and my brain felt like mush. Every once in a while, I'd try to lay down for a quick nap. But my body was too wired to fall asleep, and I would just lay there, thinking about the other things on my to-do list. So, I'd get up and start moving again, pouring myself another cup of coffee to get through the slump. Sometimes I'd make myself put on a workout video and do a second workout to wake myself up… and try to lose those last fifteen pounds that I was constantly worried about.

This is the reality I lived for fifteen years, all the way into perimenopause. I thought exercise was the most important way to work on my figure and manage my stress. It was my "me time," and heaven knows I didn't get much of that. I loved the high I would get from exercise, although it only lasted a short period of time before I crashed.

The more I studied women's hormones and the more I worked with women in the perimenopausal stage of life, the more I realized that pushing exercise onto a body that was already stressed out was one of the worst things women could do in their forties.

## Cardiovascular Exercise and Cortisol

Many of the women I worked with had a similar addiction to cardiovascular ("cardio") exercise. **Cardio** refers to activities that increase both heart rate and respiration while at the same time utilizing large muscle groups rhythmically and repetitively—activities like jogging, group exercise classes, and using machines like the stair climber, treadmill, or exercise bike.

When heart rate and respiration are elevated, our old friend cortisol comes out to play. In the short term, cortisol can increase energy and lower fatigue (1). This makes exercise feel good for a period of time. This is why working out hard, going for a run, or completing a HIIT class can feel so amazing for a while. Cortisol is a steroid, and steroids can make us feel pretty fantastic.

It's not just cortisol that is involved in the hormonal response to exercise. The stress hormones adrenaline and noradrenaline, along with inflammation-inducing chemical messengers called cytokines, are released during exercise itself (2). As exercise intensity increases, more stress is placed on the endocrine system, which leads to greater disturbances in our hormones (3). High-intensity exercise combined with inadequate recovery and nutrition can cause declines in estrogen, progesterone, and testosterone levels, and can also cause disturbances in cortisol. When I run the Dried Urine Test for Comprehensive Hormones (DUTCH) on a client and I see a pattern of low estrogen, low progesterone, low testosterone, and low cortisol, I can fairly accurately predict that she has a pattern of **Overexercising** combined with **Over-dieting**.

This can mean trouble, especially in perimenopause. Even women who exercise daily can begin to gain weight in their forties. As women gain a few pounds here and there, seemingly out of nowhere, they fall into the trap of trying to exercise even more and eating even less. Researchers at Penn State University found that cutting calories by an average of about 600 calories a day compared to **baseline** needs over just three menstrual cycles is enough to throw off a woman's period (5).

# Baseline Calorie Needs

*What is baseline?* A moderately active woman should eat around 2,000 calories each day just to maintain normal body function (6). At 2,000 calories a day, a woman should sleep well, enjoy balanced moods, experience healthy libido, grow strong hair and nails, have plenty of energy, and digest her meals well enough to have a healthy bowel movement every day. But because most women have trained themselves since adolescence to cut calories and food in order to lose weight (one study showed that on average, women spent 17 years of their lives dieting), very few women are actually eating enough to fuel their bodies (7). Of course, we don't have accurate data on this, as even dietitians tend to underestimate and under-report their daily calorie intake (8).

When I have my clients use a food tracking app to track their food for a few weeks, I see everything from an average of 900 to 3,200 calories a day. Very few women naturally land at the 2,000-calorie average mark. *Our collective minds and bodies have been so confused by diet culture that we have no idea what we should actually be eating.*

Over 88% of people who try to lose weight combine exercise with food restriction, so it's likely that you've tried this pairing multiple times over the course of your life (9). This is an Over: **Over-dieting**.

If a woman is under baseline, adding extra exercise in yet another attempt to lose weight, she might end up with a cumulative calorie deficit of about 600 calories. That's enough to disturb her menstrual cycle and her hormones. In fact, women who exercise too much have lower levels of the hormones we need to have normal periods, specifically luteinizing hormone, prolactin, and estradiol-17 beta (10).

Are you looking at your wearable fitness tracker constantly throughout the day, trying to determine your "calorie burn" for that day and hoping that you'll be in a deficit? Do you wonder why this math stops checking out in perimenopause? And are you suffering from more fatigue, injury, pain, and illness after exercise than you experienced in your 20s and 30s?

# The Physical Effects of Overexercise

The same exercise class you enjoyed without repercussions a few years ago can now be a source of regular exposure to stress hormones. This can increase the negative health effects of chronic stress. Exercise-induced pain, exhaustion, and injury can also induce psychological stress, which can cause insomnia, irritability, and mood swings. During exercise, the body also increases the production of reactive oxygen species, which are inflammatory substances that can impair some immune cell functions and lead to more frequent infections (do you notice yourself getting sicker more often than you used to?) (11).

**Gut permeability** is the intestinal lining's ability to control what passes through it into the rest of the body. A healthy gut is semi-permeable, allowing nutrients to pass through while keeping out harmful substances. However, some people have increased intestinal permeability (also known as "leaky gut"), which means their guts allow more than nutrients and water to pass through. Gut permeability increases during heavy exercise, which can indirectly increase food sensitivities and contribute to the development of "leaky gut." This can cause intestinal issues like inflammatory bowel disease (IBD) and irritable bowel syndrome (IBS) as well as irritable liver disease, alcoholic liver disease, nonalcoholic fatty liver disease, steatohepatitis, liver cirrhosis, collagen diseases, and even diabetes mellitus (12).

# Ancestral Wisdom

Your great-great-great-great grandmother likely wasn't doing any intentional cardio exercise. In fact, aerobic exercise wasn't even performed for its own sake until 1968 (13). Up until then, functional exercise had been part of human existence, although it was not separate from normal daily activities. People didn't "work out." Movement was necessary for life, and your ancestor knew she had to be physically strong to carry children, care for farm animals, lift heavy things, and walk for long distances without difficulty. She would never have gotten up before dawn to "go for a jog." To quote Grandma Frances in the movie *Christmas Vacation* out of context: "*I hope you kids see what a silly waste of resources this was.*"

Your ancestor needed to allocate energy to the things that mattered, like caring for her family, preparing food, and taking care of the home. Now that many women are doing all of these things and *also* working outside the home, it becomes even more important for us to not waste our limited energy resources.

Heaping stress hormone-inducing exercise on a body that is already stuck in fight-or-flight mode will not give us the results we are looking for in our perimenopausal stage. But movement is still important. Instead of trying *harder*, now is the time to try *different*.

# The Power of Walking

The simple act of walking is a powerful tool for function and fitness. In 2020, I ran a free online challenge for women (14). I asked women to walk 10,000 steps a day, outside, every day for seven days. This is the equivalent of about five miles. Getting in this much walking is neither easy nor intuitive! However, I had 213 women join that challenge. I polled the women at the end of the week to ask them about their experience. Listen to what some of my formerly sedentary clients had to say about daily walking:

Amy thought she was pretty active. But when she started tracking her steps, here's what she had to say: "I'm pretty active on the exercise front but apparently very sedentary in terms of walking (also I just don't tend to carry my phone with me), but I made it to above 7,000 on Monday, 8,000 on Tuesday, and finally hit 10,000 today!"

Jacqueline, a former cardio queen, said, "[I learned] that I don't always need to do a strenuous workout to feel good."

Jessica struggled with sugar cravings and afternoon fatigue. But after starting to walk 10,000 steps a day, she reported: "When I walk more, I have more energy and [fewer] chocolate/sweet cravings."

Jennifer had a three-year-old son and never felt like she recovered her body after childbirth. She also had a hard time sleeping at night. But she committed to walking regularly with our group. After a few weeks, she wrote, "Since I have had my son, I am sadly out of shape. But I have noticed since I have focused on getting my 10,000 steps in a day, I sleep better at night."

Whitney was active in the CrossFit community and really loved her workout days. But on the days that she did not include a run, she realized she was fairly sedentary. She said, "On days when I don't run, my step count is pretty low, even if I walk the dog. I need to make more of an effort to be active on those days." Whitney continued to suffer from increasingly frustrating perimenopause symptoms until we started working together privately. You'll hear more about her story in Chapter 10.

Wendy worked at a desk all day and got sick of sitting in a chair, on the computer for hours on end. Walking was a new habit that gave her a physical and mental break from her computer. She told our group, "I enjoy walking. I like that it forces me to take a break from work."

Like so many of us, these women are busy, working moms. I asked them to carve out about one hour a day to devote to functional movement and overall health. It wasn't easy for many of them to initiate this new habit, but once they began working on walking 10,000 steps a day, they realized it was something they wanted to do long term.

Julie and Stephanie were addicted to heavy cardiovascular exercise, claiming it helped them manage stress. During the walking challenge, I invited my ladies to step back from the cortisol-inducing heavy cardio exercise and simply walk. Both ladies reported positive results. Julie said, "I learned that I don't have to kill myself with vigorous workouts every day. Walking 30 minutes or more a day at a rapid pace, about 103 steps a minute, will help my hormones stay in check and keep me healthy."

Stephanie said, "Just walking IS good exercise. *Walking is enough.*" (15)

Walking is my therapy. My sister Jessie and I are neighbors and best friends. We make it a priority to catch up with each other over our weekly walks. Getting fresh air, sunshine, and a good talk session leaves both of us feeling better. Jessie is a gifted tennis player and is on the court almost every single day, but she always has energy to meet me for a walk and talk therapy session. It's definitely a highlight of my week.

# The Research on Walking

The research backs up what we girls have experienced. One study asked women who previously walked around 5,000 steps a day (the national average) to walk 10,000 steps a day. The study found that participants experienced less anxiety, depression, anger, confusion, fatigue, and total mood distress. They also had statistically significant decreases in body weight, BMI, waist circumference, and body fat percentage after walking ≥10,000 steps daily for twelve weeks (16).

Happier *and* fitter? Yes, please! I find that for my clients, walking 10,000 steps a day is good. But walking 10,000 steps a day *outside* is great. Exercise in nature has been associated with lower cortisol, heart rate, blood pressure, blood glucose, and cholesterol, as well as lower fatigue and negative emotions. It can also contribute to higher energy levels (17).

If you're already walking 10,000 steps a day and you're trying to lose weight, make sure you've optimized your diet by getting enough protein and calories, and then increase your steps to 15,000 steps a day. I haven't seen a lot of benefit in going over that 15,000-step mark. I've noticed that women get hungrier at that level of steps. The sweet spot seems to be 10,000 to 15,000 steps a day, six to seven days a week. It can also help people get off the treadmill and get outside.

# Strength Training Essentials

The second exercise that's helpful in perimenopause is **strength training**. Don't overthink this. Get yourself some weights and slowly start lifting them, heavier and heavier. I recommend finding a knowledgeable personal trainer in your area for advice. I myself have worked with a few on-line trainers, and while it's convenient, it's not as effective as working out with the in-person supervision of a professional.

If you can't afford a professional, look up videos online about how to start strength training. You can always start with bodyweight exercises. I'll have some clients do ten pushups, ten sit-ups, ten squats, and ten lunges right after waking up if they are brand new to strength training. I also recommend the excellent app "Stronger by the Day" for home and gym-based workouts (18).

Your ancestor needed her body to be strong and fit in order to do all of the things she had to do each day. You're no different. We need our bodies to be functional for as long as possible. If you think you're too old or too out of shape, check out the Train with Joan Instagram account (@trainwithjoan) for some inspiration (19). She definitely inspires me!

# The Research on Strength Training

Research highlights the importance of strength training for women in midlife. One study showed that women in peri-menopause had greater fat mass, less muscle, and a greater percentage of body fat compared to pre- and postmenopausal women. Yes, you're reading that right. Belly fat among the perimenopausal women averaged 16% higher than among their premenopausal counterparts and 5% higher than the postmenopausal women in the study. The authors concluded, "Perimenopause may be the most opportune window for lifestyle intervention, as this group experienced the onset of unfavorable body composition and metabolic characteristics". Interestingly, the perimenopausal women in this study also ate lower amounts of protein, or 64 grams a day. The premenopausal women ate 71 grams, and the postmenopausal women ate 67 grams. The researchers determined that perimenopausal women can avoid muscle loss and slow metabolism by engaging in activities that help to maintain muscle mass and fat-burning capacity, such as strength training (20).

Strength training and walking tend to be the magic movement combination for women in perimenopause. I see it all the time. Just walking and lifting weights will help to reduce stress, get out of fight-or-flight mode, and achieve the body composition you want in your forties and beyond. Your great-great-great-great grandchildren will be looking to *you* for inspiration.

## How To Exercise Differently in Perimenopause

Exercise becomes simple in perimenopause. Cancel your gym membership and spend that money on a facial or a massage. Sell your Peloton and invest in a sauna bag. Get rid of your treadmill and purchase some heavy weights. You'll feel calm, fit, and strong by adopting this routine.

## Exercise Action Items

There are two things you need to do for exercise, and two things only:

1. **Walk 10,000 to 15,000 steps a day outside.** Start with "exercise snacks," walking for just fifteen minutes at a time, two to three times a day. Track your steps with an inexpensive pedometer, your phone, or a fitness tracker. Every fifteen minutes of walking equates to roughly 1,500 steps. As you get stronger, walk for thirty minutes, two to three times a day. Work up to about ninety minutes of walking total, spaced throughout the day.
   **Bonus points:** Get yourself a best friend/sister to do "therapy walks" with!
2. **Lift heavy weights two to three times a week for thirty to forty-five minutes.** Find a trainer in your area, ask a knowledgeable friend, use the app I mentioned called "Stronger By The Day," or look up videos online that teach you how to lift weights.

If you get 10,000 steps a day and begin a slow and steady weight training routine, you'll enjoy a strong body and a reasonable weight while protect your hormones.

CHAPTER 5:

# Banishing Over-Stress – Healing Can't Happen When You're Stuck in Fight-or-Flight Mode

IT'S HARD TO have an Easy Perimenopause when you're stuck in fight-or-flight mode. A nervous system that's constantly on high alert can cause a wide variety of symptoms to creep up in perimenopause.

Many women report not *feeling* stressed out. Yet when they step back and look at their schedule, they realize that their days are set up to keep them in a constant state of stress.

### *Kristy*

Kristy laughed.

> *"An Epsom salt bath? I don't have time for that. I've got five kids and I homeschool. I barely have time to sneak off to the bathroom."*

Like so many women, Kristy loved the thrill of implementing new diets. Changing her nutrition felt empowering and doable. Besides, she'd been told her whole life that dieting would help her lose weight and feel better. She was a diet pro! But when I encouraged her to recognize that nutritional optimization is only a part of a true hormonal health puzzle, she worried that she might not have enough time to focus on anything other than diet as she tried to care for her large family. Homeschooling kept her busy and on edge, and Kristy was constantly exhausted, needing naps almost daily. She felt wired most of the day, quickly moving from one activity to the next, only to fall into bed exhausted at the end of the day.

Yet after just four weeks of implementing stress-management practices like Epsom salt baths, Kristy started to feel very differently. She pushed into the stress management part of the program. Soon her hormones began to regulate, her energy increased, and her skin began looking better. She spent more time outside each day and noticed that as her kids followed suit, they also began experiencing the benefits of sleep.

> "I hit all the goals today. In the past, I would always skip the sun, salt baths, and workouts. So, I'm pretty proud of myself. And I'm quite pleased to see that when I walk for an hour, it's so easy to hit that 10,000 goal.
>
> "This last period was super light with very small clots. I remember how you mentioned that this means extra estrogen is leaving my body. I'm surprised at how much energy I have in wanting to get out and walk. It's like I want to move my body. It doesn't feel like a chore. I'm not crashing around that two o'clock period. If the house is quiet, I'll choose to relax on the couch and nap. But the few times I've done that, taking a less than twenty-minute nap is more than

*enough and I'm up and ready. In the past, I would take the full two-hour nap my kids took and still want more sleep as I dragged myself out of bed.*

*"More people are noticing my clear skin. My kids are even starting to wake up earlier. I'm not sure why, but maybe it's because we are being more intentional [about getting] outside and their internal clocks are changing. It seems like they are falling asleep better now that they are getting to run around outside."*

## Leanne

Leanne struggled with seasonal mood imbalances. She was a California girl, through and through, but had recently relocated to a rainy state. If she wasn't intentional about getting outside and spending time in the sun, her mood started to deteriorate. As part of my programs, I ask my ladies to spend at least thirty minutes a day outside. Many of them notice positive changes in their mood and sleep. Leanne was no different. She was in an **Over—Overstress**.

*"I forget how lack of sunshine affects my mood. It's been overcast and raining this last week, which has left me feeling glum. But the moment the sun comes out I feel loads better."*

During the course of our time together, Leanne worked on being mindful of her commitments to herself and others. As a busy mom, overscheduling became a regular occurrence. That busyness often crowded out healthy activities, like preparing healthy food, spending time outdoors, and taking an Epsom salt bath at the end of each day. But when we spent a concentrated month together in a group coaching setting, Leanne was able to be intentional about incorporating these stress management strategies into her day. And her mood and outlook improved considerably.

> *"I have learned that it is about balance. That's not something new for me, but I easily forget to balance myself and my life, and that's where the problems pop up for me. I know I can't do it all, but when I can find a happy medium in all things, I feel so much better."*

## Lynn

Just like the rest of my busy clients, Lynn tended to overextend herself to serve her family, friends, and colleagues. But as we focused on intentional rest over the course of a month, she realized that she could not neglect taking care of herself and setting boundaries.

> *"Today, I learned that it's okay to say no. I don't need to feel bad about it, and my body will thank me for not overextending myself."*

These are all real women who elected to spend a month with me learning the importance of eating more protein, spending sufficient time in the sun, taking Epsom salt baths, and walking 10,000 steps a day. When you practice the basics consistently, the body naturally slips out of fight-or-flight mode and the nervous system begins to balance. It's at this point that sleep gets deeper, the weight falls off, and mood stabilizes.

## Learning to Manage Stress

One of the basics is *learning how to manage stress.* I used to try to help clients remove stress from their lives. In my mind, if the stressor was not there, life would be easier and consequently, the autonomic nervous system would naturally balance out. But the more women I worked with, the more I realized that nearly every woman lives a pretty darn stressful life, and there is no way to remove all of our problems in life on this side of heaven.

I also started realizing that it's not necessarily *valuable* for the body to remove all stressors. A little bit of stress can help our bodies and brains grow stronger. Finding a way to manage these stressors without letting them overwhelm your brain and body is important. In this chapter, I'll teach you the exact ways I help women successfully manage their stress levels and experience deeper resilience and contentment.

## Stress and Hormones

Stress and hormones are integrally connected. Even minimal stress can activate the hypothalamic-pituitary-adrenal (HPA) axis, which in turn activates several different hormone-secreting systems (1). When researchers examined the consequences of stress on the brain, they discovered alarming structural changes like a reduction in brain mass. This means the brain actually shrinks in size when we are under prolonged stress! The brain is our commander-in-chief, managing everything from heart rate to mood regulation. When the brain starts to atrophy, the body can quickly follow suit (2). This explains a lot for perimenopausal women who complain of increasing brain fog, forgetfulness, and mood swings. A stress-induced shrinking brain may be to blame.

For perimenopausal women, natural fluctuations in hormonal balance on top of stress-induced brain changes can cause irritability, anger, mood swings, brain fog, and in the long term, it can even contribute to the development of certain neurodegenerative diseases. When stress signals are sent to the brain via an organ called the hypothalamus, another organ called the pituitary gland sends signals to the adrenal glands to release cortisol. Due to its lipophilic properties, which mean that it easily diffuses through fats, cortisol can cross the blood-brain barrier. Once inside the brain, hormones like cortisol can cause alterations in the function and structure of our brain's nerve cells, interfering with memory, concentration, and other crucial cognitive functions. The hypothalamus and adrenal glands also have a strong influence on the ovaries and the thyroid. *This is why periods, sleep, mood, and weight can all become very problematic for the chronically stressed woman.*

I regularly tell my clients that their bodies *simply cannot heal* if they are stuck in this stress response.

Let's explore the real experiences of Michelle, Lori, and Anne. These quick case studies illustrate how chronic stress can have profound and diverse effects on the systems of the body.

## Symptoms of Chronic Stress

In perimenopause, symptoms of chronic stress can present in a variety of ways that are not normally attributed to hormones. I want to introduce you to a few more of my wonderful clients and illustrate how stress can cause strange symptoms to pop up:

### *Michelle*

As a POP Pilates Advanced instructor, Michelle has been teaching Pilates and yoga for years. In fact, she was recently a featured instructor on the new POP Pilates Presenter Team's video series. While Michelle's body is flexible and strong, she also battles chronic pain from both scoliosis and a childhood accident. Michelle has busy days, often hosting her young adult sons, traveling with her husband, picking up extra work, and serving on the lay counseling team at her church. Her pain was constant, and she often battled crippling morning depression. She knew from experience that if she just made it to lunchtime, the dark cloud of the morning would lift and she would be able to get through her day.

Michelle went from practitioner to practitioner, seeking relief from her pain, insomnia, and mood issues. She slowly accumulated a supplement regimen of almost forty pills a day. But the pain and mood issues persisted, and at night, she rarely slept for more than two hours at a time.

When Michelle and I had our first call, I learned she was only eating one meal a day. She usually fasted until dinner, fueling herself with coffee throughout the rest of the day. After her last class, she would eat a healthy dinner. But soon after her meal, she often found herself snacking on popcorn, chips, wine, and chocolate until bedtime. With a perfect Pilates body, Michelle wasn't worried about her weight. However, she was eager to get relief from her pain and insomnia.

Michelle immediately began to eat regular nourishing meals, but we also had work to do on her stress management. She began getting morning sun. She continued her quiet time with God each morning. She started practicing breathing exercises. She also wrestled with cutting back on her teaching schedule, as she slowly realized that hours of exercise each day had depleted her body of cortisol. When we tested her cortisol levels, they were below the low end of the reference range on the DUTCH. Studies have shown that low cortisol levels are associated with chronic pain, and Michelle's low levels were a clear contributing factor to her daily neck, shoulder, and scalp pain (3, 4).

After four months of working together, Michelle made significant strides in her mood and pain management. Here's what she had to say:

> *"For YEARS my body had been giving me feedback clues about the toxicity of my stress levels, but I just didn't understand. I wanted so badly to do all the right things and my body was working so hard to keep up with my demands. The really tragic part is that the harder I pushed and the more I fought to keep it all together, the sicker I became. Obviously, there's very little in life that we can control, but in a very real sense, I did this to me. I still struggle with a lot of guilt and honestly, I don't even know that I can articulate what it is that I feel so darn guilty about.*
>
> *"I (now have) permission to laugh at myself and give myself grace. It's a mental and physical space that I didn't have for myself before."*

## Lori

Lori is a busy mother of eight and grandmother to many young grandchildren. She doesn't look like your typical grandmother—spry and full of life, her long dark hair is always perfectly done and her infectious laugh sounds more like a teenager's than a nana's. She homeschools her children and travels often to visit her family in other states. She loves to cook and clean and babysit her grandchildren, wanting nothing more than to love and serve her family well. But the constant travel and work came at a price: her gut was constantly distressed.

Lori's frustrating bowel issues highlight yet another victim of stress—the digestive system. Stress can alter gut motility, increase inflammation, and even change the composition of the gut microbiome, leaving the body more susceptible to gastrointestinal disorders. By eating regular meals, getting enough protein, and working on stress management techniques like deep breathing, time in the sauna, and getting to bed before 11 p.m., Lori saw almost immediate improvements in her gut health.

## *Anne*

Anne is Italian. She loves her bread, pasta, and sweets. Her regular extended family gatherings always include plenty of traditional Italian food. Anne homeschools her three boys and works long days in the home and the schoolroom. She has always been active in her church, often hosting events for nearly 100 teenagers at the home she shares with her husband, Nate. The couple also participates in the counseling ministry at church and enjoys traveling together when Nate's company sends him on work trips.

With her jam-packed schedule, Anne rarely had time to decompress. Emotionally, this didn't seem to bother her. If you meet her in real life, she is always cheerful and gracious. But physically, her body was fed up. Anne started experiencing terrifying monthly hemorrhaging, losing so much blood during her period that she would have to lie in bed for a few days each month to recover.

When we started working together, we found that her estrogen and progesterone levels were perfectly normal. But when we ran a stool test and a food sensitivity test, we found that she was highly sensitive to gluten, a protein found in wheat, sugar, soy, and corn. Anne had been eating these foods regularly, especially gluten. She loved her Italian wheat bread and wheat pasta! The foods that Anne was sensitive to were significant stressors to her body, keeping her in a state of fight-or-flight every time she ate them.

We immediately put together a strategy for removing these foods from Anne's diet. She was game for anything, desperate for relief from the awful periods she had been suffering from. After removing the foods she was sensitive to, eating significantly more protein, cutting out sugar, and getting to bed earlier, Anne had a perfectly normal period in less than two months. Here's what she said,

> *"I started my period and it has been pretty 'normal.' Heavy for the first two days, medium for the next two days, and light today. No cramping. Praise the Lord! No clots!"*

Michelle, Lori, and Anne are real women—valued and beloved clients that I became quite close to over our months of intensive work together. Their stories illustrate the ways that stress can manifest in real life, particularly during the perimenopausal years. The physical symptoms that often crop up in perimenopause aren't always simply hormonal in nature—chronic pain, gut issues, and period problems can all be symptoms of perimenopause, and these symptoms are absolutely exacerbated by stress. Understanding the link between stress and its bodily effects allows women can proactively address these challenges and use the strategies below to mitigate stress and promote a healthier transition through perimenopause.

# Practical Tips for Managing Stress

Managing stress does not come easily to women in their forties, overburdened and overwhelmed with the responsibilities of work, family, and life. You've likely heard the axiom "What's measured can be managed." Measuring stress response can be a useful tool in the battle against stress. I like to have clients track something called **heart rate variability (HRV)** when we start working together so they can get a visual of what their stress levels look like throughout the day and night. Using heart rate variability as a personal diagnostic tool to manage stress has been one of the most helpful resources for my Type-A, overachieving, result-oriented clients.

HRV refers to the time variation between consecutive heartbeats, serving as a measurement of the autonomic nervous system's response to internal and external stressors. High HRV is a sign that your body can adapt well to changes. It means your body is responding properly to both the sympathetic and parasympathetic nervous system. Low HRV can indicate that your body is having trouble adapting to changes and may be struggling with current or future health issues.

Heart rate variability is different from **heart rate**, which simply refers to the number of times your heart beats every minute. A high heart rate isn't necessarily a good thing, as it can mean the body is stressed. However, high HRV is a really good thing! It means that your body is resilient and manages stress well.

For perimenopausal women, fluctuations in hormone levels can significantly impact the autonomic nervous system. This can lead to changes in HRV. A higher HRV often indicates a healthier, more resilient cardiovascular system that's capable of adaptively responding to life's stressors. A lower HRV is associated with stress, fatigue, and even an increased risk for cardiovascular diseases.

Think of HRV as the rhythm of a woman's day, constantly changing with each new activity and demand—in some moments it's lively and free-flowing, while at other times, it's more rigid and structured.

Imagine HRV as the back-and-forth dance of a typical busy day:

- **High HRV** is like the early morning after a restful sleep when the kids are still in bed, and you're savoring a quiet cup of tea—a moment when your body feels open and ready for anything. A high HRV indicates your body's resilience and ability to adapt to different situations, thanks to activities that recharge your energy, like a balanced workout or mindfulness practice.
- **Low HRV** mirrors the frenzied rush of the carpool and of juggling work emails with preparing dinner amidst the chaos of homework and bedtime routines. At these times, your body is more focused on handling immediate tasks, leaving less room for flexibility. Stress, lack of sleep, or skipping meals can cause this dip in variability—similar to how a hectic day can drain your energy.

## Measuring HRV

While there are many devices that are able to measure HRV, I like to have my clients use a device called an Oura Ring. This wearable technology gives us excellent insights into not only HRV, but also sleep and movement.

By observing HRV through the use of something like the Oura Ring (or Apple Watch or Whoop strap), we can gain real-time feedback on bodies' reactions to stress. With that information, we can tailor stress management techniques and lifestyle adjustments to increase overall well-being during the stressors of perimenopause. For example, if your HRV is consistently low for days or weeks on end, we know that you'll likely need to back off on your busy schedule. You may need to cut down on the amount of exercise you're doing, get to bed earlier, take more Epsom salt baths, or engage in regular breathwork. You may need more calories. Either way, the measurement is there, and now it can be managed.

## Managing HRV

HRV can be a wonderful way to observe the stress patterns of your life. However, if you can't afford or don't want to use a device, you can simply start breathing differently during times of stress. When we inhale, our heart rate increases. When we exhale, our heart rate decreases. During times of stress, it can be beneficial to focus on *breathing out*—the act of simply exhaling for as long as or longer than our inhale can be a powerful tool to get out of fight-or-flight mode and feel less stressed and more balanced. In fact, one study showed that a prolonged exhale significantly increased mood and decreased stress even more than meditation (5).

Take heart, fellow Type As! If you feel like you're ill-equipped to meditate, just start spending one minute a day breathing in for three seconds through your nose and breathing out for seven seconds through your mouth. In fact, *stop reading and try this activity right now.* Come back in five minutes and notice how much calmer you feel.

This is one of the major coping strategies I encourage my clients to use. Adults generally take about fifteen breaths each minute. Slowing your breath rate down to six breaths per minute can increase feelings of peacefulness, decrease anxiety, reduce mind-wandering and intrusive thoughts, and even increase reaction time and problem-solving (6). This means that when you're spending time practicing your breathwork, you become more focused and less agitated. This is a great trade-off for spending a few minutes a day practicing breathing techniques.

I'm a fan of breathwork because I like to take an active part in my stress management, and I can tell that my nervous system is more balanced when I complete this exercise daily. Most of my clients see an immediate improvement in stress levels with this one simple hack, too. Elisa reported,

*"I can now walk away from stressful situations at times and just go breathe. I can say I am much more balanced now. I also am quicker to recognize when I'm stressed, whereas before, I had just learned to carry it and not listen to my body's warning signals."*

## Three Breathing Techniques

### 1. Deep Breathing

- Breathe in through the nose for three seconds.
- Breathe out through the mouth for seven seconds.
- Repeat six times.

## 2. Box Breathing

- Breathe in through the nose for three seconds.
- Hold for three seconds.
- Breathe out through the mouth for three seconds.
- Hold for three seconds.
- Repeat five times.

## 3. The 4-2-6 Method

- Breathe in through the nose for four seconds.
- Hold for two seconds.
- Breathe out through the mouth for six seconds.
- Repeat five times.

# Emotional and Spiritual Stress: My Story

Sure, there's a physical component to stress. But as women, we also know that there are mental, emotional, and even spiritual components to stress. I practice all of the physical stress-reducing principles that I'm sharing in this book. But for me, the spiritual component is just as important. When I used to strive *so hard* to do all of the things by myself, I felt empty and inadequate. But around age twenty, I became a Christian and I started realizing that I didn't have to try to measure up all on my own. I realized that God's grace was sufficient for me. I love the words of Ruth Chou Simons in her book When Strivings Cease:

*"After years and years of striving, I simply wore out. I had a full-on case of striving fatigue."*

If you resonate with that, check out her book. It's a fantastic resource for "replacing the gospel of self-improvement with the gospel of life-transforming grace."

When I began to really learn what it meant to care for myself well so that I could care well for those who depended on me—*my family!*—I had to do a lot of uncomfortable things. I stopped bringing dinners to families in need. For years, I would cook two meals and then strap my four tiny kids into a car at dinner time and drive across town to bring a meal to a family who had just had a baby, or who had an illness in the family. I would yell at my kids, cry while driving, plaster a fake smile on my face as I dropped off the meal, trudge back home to feed my cranky and confused kids, and finally collapse into bed, unable to fall asleep due to my elevated cortisol levels. One day, I just stopped signing up for meal trains. I stopped volunteering in the church nursery. I got tired of dreading Sunday mornings where I would skip the soul-nourishing time of being in God's Word with my church family and instead spend two hours with my own four small children plus another twenty-five small children. I wanted to perform, to please, and to perfect. And then one day, I just couldn't. I too had a full-on case of striving fatigue, as it were.

I'm not saying I never serve anymore. I do! My husband Beau and I love to serve. I just do it from an open and willing heart when I'm actually able to do it, instead of giving God and people my leftovers with a side of martyrdom and bitterness. The service is much more fulfilling now.

You don't have to do it all. Take care of yourself with the basic principles you're learning here and use that extra energy and vigor to serve your family and husband first. When your primary responsibilities are fulfilled, you can move on to serving a bigger circle. Trust me, this shift will be so helpful.

## Baths and Stress Management

Let's switch topics and visit my all-time favorite stress-reducing practice: the bath. We discussed baths in a previous chapter, but baths are so amazing for stress management that I want to expand on this information a bit more.

There's a reason why the term "spa" is associated with rest and indulgence. In fact, the word *spa* is an acronym for the Latin phrase *Salus per Aquam*, meaning "health from water" (7). One bath historian wrote, "The Roman Baths are so fundamental to our modern understanding of baths that a whole city is named after them. Unlike many public baths at the time, these baths featured a naturally heated, larger area for actual swimming, not just soaking. There was also a 'dry sweating room' and a series of plunge pools" (8). The rhythms of our ancestors offer so much wisdom—since bathing was a necessary part of life, why not make it as relaxing and enjoyable as possible?

Investing in a massage or facial regularly can be a powerful stress-busting hack, but many of us can't afford a weekly spa treatment.

However, many of us can absolutely block off thirty minutes each evening for an Epsom salt bath: a mini spa in the privacy of your own home. Epsom salt baths are one of the best ways to literally soak away the stress of the day and physiologically prepare your body for sleep.

Epsom salt baths are easy. Buy a large bag of Epsom salts. Run a bath as hot as you can stand it and add three cups of salts to the bath. Sometimes I'll add eight to ten drops of a relaxing essential oil like lavender or rose. If I'm feeling under the weather, I'll add eucalyptus oil.

Ease into the tub and stay in the water for at least ten minutes, or until you feel hot and start sweating. This is the time for you to decompress, so keep phones and screens far away from your soak. Your great-great-great grandmother wasn't watching TV in the tub!

Once you're warm and a little sweaty, wet a washcloth with cold water and place it on the back of your neck. It will feel amazing. Carefully get out of the tub. I like to spread a towel on my bathroom floor and lie down on the towel, covering myself with another towel. I do this until I've stopped sweating and I'm ready to finish my bedtime preparations of applying lotion and getting into my pajamas.

*A gentle reminder: Use good judgment. Don't get in a bath that is too hot, and don't get in a bath if you're dehydrated or under the influence of drugs or alcohol. Be careful not to slip. Call for help if you feel disoriented.*

For overall health and stress management, bathing trumps the shower every time. In fact, after immersion in 104-degree Fahrenheit water, participants in one study reported less stress, tension, anxiety, anger, hostility, and depression (9). Immersion bathing can actually decrease fatigue (10). Study participants even reported smiling more while in a bath. This is likely because immersion bathing increases blood flow, providing more oxygen and nutrients to tissues. Increased circulation increases deep body temperature, which gets you out of fight-or-flight mode and activates the parasympathetic nervous system.

The gentle increase in heart rate during a hot bath also increases blood oxygen and decreases blood carbon dioxide, which can actually increase metabolism and eliminate waste products. This means that taking regular baths can help you feel happier and can also increase your fat-burning abilities. Taking hot baths up to three times a week is also associated with better immune function (11). Baths aren't just for when you're sick—they're for preventing illness in the first place!

## Stress Management and the Vagus Nerve

Once you've mastered breathing and baths, you can move on to managing stress by activating your vagus nerve. This is an incredibly useful skill. As you start activating this healing power, you'll realize that you are more in control of your health than you ever thought you were. And that's a great feeling.

The vagus nerve (from the Latin meaning "to wander") is a sensory nerve and the longest cranial nerve in the body. It starts at the base of the brain, travels down both sides of the neck and the heart, throughout the stomach area, and into the intestines.

Like a muscle, the vagus nerve can be toned and strengthened. It performs the following tasks:

- Keeps the larynx open for breathing
- Slows/regulates the heartbeat
- Stimulates the secretion of saliva, release of bile, and peristalsis (contraction) of the bowels
- Contracts the bladder
- Sends messages to the brain to produce/release oxytocin (the feel-good/bonding hormone)
- Reduces anxiety and depression

- Reduces stress and inflammation
- Increases immunity and longevity

When the vagus nerve is not sending or receiving the correct signals, it can become underactive. An underactive vagus nerve can cause imbalances in functions like heartbeat, digestion, bonding, mood, inflammation, and immunity. A common cause of an underactive vagus nerve is chronic stress (12).

Stress doesn't need to "feel" like stress. In fact, I have many clients who tell me that they don't feel stressed. But when we run a functional lab test like the DUTCH (a hormone test), their sky-high cortisol levels tell a different story. Stress can come from the outside—difficult relationships, financial hardships, a tough job, or parenting teenagers. Stress can also come from the inside—food sensitivities, recurrent infections like Epstein-Barr virus, micronutrient deficiencies like too little dietary potassium, an autoimmune burden, or chronic inflammation.

All of these things can keep your body in fight-or-flight mode. But the purpose of this chapter is to give you tools to help you ditch that mode and relax into a more balanced state.

# Practical Ways to Care for Your Vagus Nerve

You can start working on vagus nerve health with these exercises:

- **Gargling**: Gargling vigorously with water after you brush your teeth every morning can really strengthen your vagus nerve. This improves movement in your di-

gestive tract and can really help with constipation and a
sluggish bowel. Plus, it's kind of fun.

- **Chanting, humming, and singing**: Singing out loud,
  chanting, and humming also activate the vagus nerve.
  Next time you're in your car, sing as loud as you can! I
  was not blessed with a good singing voice, so I opt to
  hum in the car. But I do this regularly.

- **Cold exposure**: This one's not for you if you're actively
  stuck in fight-or-flight mode and every little thing caus-
  es you distress. If you're feeling too overwhelmed and
  vulnerable, don't worry about cold exposure just yet.
  But if you're feeling stronger, eating plenty of protein,
  getting good sleep, and walking outside in nature, consider a little bit of daily cold exposure. Here's how to do
  it: At the end of your hot shower, simply turn the hot
  water off and stand in the cold water for ten to thirty
  seconds. Let the water cascade down your face, head,
  and neck. If you can go longer than thirty seconds,
  that's even better. If you want to get out of the shower
  after the cold spray, do so. If you want to turn the hot
  water on again and warm up a bit before stepping out,
  that's fine too! You will feel so good after this little hit
  of cold exposure—it becomes addictive.

A variety of stress management techniques are included
in this chapter so that you can pick a few that resonate with
you. Choose two to begin implementing this week. Can you
commit to taking a nightly Epsom salt bath and including
five minutes of deep breathing as you sink into your hot
bath? Or would you rather work on your vagus nerve for
the next seven days, gargling and singing as you brush your
teeth each morning? What would help you manage stress

most effectively? Find activities that work for your schedule and your disposition and begin to practice these new habits.

## Stress Management Action Items

- Prioritize sleep hygiene for better quality rest. I recommend turning off all screens by 9 p.m. at the latest. Every evening, try to take a hot Epsom salt bath with three cups of bath salts and the essential oils of your choice. Once your body temperature has decreased a bit, you'll be ready for bed!

- Engage in regular physical activity appropriate for your health status. As discussed in Chapter 4, walking 10,000 steps a day (outside!) and lifting heavy weights two to three times a week should be plenty of exercise to help you get a deep night's sleep.

- Practice breathing exercises to reduce the physical impact of stress, activate your vagus nerve, and get out of fight-or-flight mode. Use a wearable device to measure HRV if desired.

- Gargle, chant, or sing for a few minutes each day to activate your vagus nerve. Deep breathing also helps activate your vagus nerve.

- Consider ending your hot shower with thirty seconds of cold water therapy.

- Get at least 100 grams of animal protein and at least 1,800 calories a day to keep your nervous system balanced.

- Treat yourself to a brand new notebook and some pretty pens and write in your journal upon before bed or waking. Spending time in concentrated reflection can help reduce anxiety.
- If stress feels unmanageable, consider stress management programs or professional help. Talking to a mental health professional or clergymember can also be helpful.

## CHAPTER 6:

# Circadian Rhythm As Your Secret Weapon Against the Overs

## *Brenda*

BRENDA IS THE CEO of a successful organic produce company. She is the happy mother of two children, one in high school and one in college. Brenda took over CEO duties for her company years ago, when the stress began to affect her health and hormones.

At the office, she was productive and confident. But her health was falling apart. After infertility issues pushed her into early menopause, she struggled with fatigue, weight gain, and lack of libido. A nasty bout of COVID-19 left her with worsened exhaustion. She was too tired to work out, and often felt like she had to choose between spending time with her family and spending time on the couch. No matter how many hours of sleep she got, Brenda still had to drag herself out of bed each morning.

After running functional lab tests that showed blood sugar management problems, high estrogen, low progesterone, extremely high cortisol, and poor estrogen clearance, she started to follow the Easy Perimenopause principles. She ate more protein, got outside more often, prioritized her sleep and rest, and balanced her hormones with specific supplements based on her lab testing. A food sensitivity test showed intolerances to milk products and coffee, so she also cut out these foods. Her new habits allowed her to get out of fight-or-flight mode and feel more like herself again.

She said, *"I have so much more energy now! And I'm smaller than my husband!"* Her dedication to working on her nutrition and stress management helped her lose twenty pounds in two months and be more present with her family.

## The Modern Disconnect

These days, it's easier than ever for women like Brenda to get to the top of their professional game. Capable, intelligent, and hardworking, Brenda easily manages a large team of people with ease and grace. But modern successes come with ancestral trade-offs. Our great-great-great grandmothers moved frequently throughout the day, spent much of their time outside, and slept when it was dark outside. Contemporary women like Brenda wake up before dawn, spend twelve hours a day inside under harsh LED lights, eat convenience meals at their desks, and sit at a computer screen for most of the day. Every aspect of the successful modern woman's circadian rhythm is a disadvantage to her hormone health. In perimenopause, this tends to catch up with her. It's important for every modern woman, CEO or not, to learn to manage her circadian rhythm.

# Circadian Rhythm

Understanding your body's natural circadian rhythm is important while managing the hormonal changes happening in perimenopause. What is the circadian rhythm? The term "circadian" comes from the Latin words *circa*, meaning "around," and *diem*, meaning "day." The circadian rhythm is the internal clock that regulates the twenty-four-hour cycle of biological processes, including sleep-wake patterns, hormone release, and metabolism.

Key hormones like cortisol, melatonin, leptin, and insulin play significant roles in this cycle. In addition to being your "stress hormone," cortisol also helps you wake up and stay alert during the day. Melatonin promotes sleep at night. Leptin signals satiety and helps regulate appetite, while insulin is essential for blood sugar control. When our circadian rhythm is altered by irregular sleep patterns or high stress, these hormones can become imbalanced, leading to issues like insomnia, weight gain, and exhaustion.

Research indicates that following natural light and dark cycles can be incredibly beneficial for managing perimenopausal symptoms. Exposure to sunlight during the day, *particularly in the morning*, is crucial for regulating your circadian rhythm. Morning sunlight tells your brain that it's time to be awake and alert, boosting cortisol levels at the appropriate time and promoting overall energy and mood. Evening darkness is equally important, as it encourages the release of melatonin, the hormone that signals your body that it's time to sleep. When we're constantly exposing ourselves to bright lights and screens after dark, our circadian hormones start to become confused.

# The Research on Circadian Rhythm

Studies suggest that disruption of these light-dark cycles can lead to many of the most frustrating perimenopausal symptoms, including sleep disturbances, mood swings, and cognitive decline. One study found that women exposed to irregular light patterns or high levels of artificial light at night experience more severe hot flashes and night sweats compared to those who maintain a natural light-dark cycle (1). This means that your morning outside time can lead to less sweaty nights!

A review highlighted the importance of circadian rhythm management in perimenopausal women, linking proper light exposure to fewer symptoms like insomnia, anxiety, and depressive moods (2). Another study showed that adhering to natural light-dark cycles decreased cognitive decline and improved mental clarity (3). Simply spending more time outdoors can improve your sleep, mood, and brain fog.

# Leptin

It's time to discuss a hormone you may not be as familiar with. **Leptin** is a hormone mainly produced by adipose (fat) cells and enterocyte cells in the small intestine. It plays a critical role in balancing energy by shutting off hunger signals. Shutting off improper hunger signals helps balance body weight.

Leptin communicates with the hypothalamus in the brain to signal that the body has enough stored energy. This signal reduces your appetite and promotes a higher metabolic rate. However, just as we can become insulin resistant, we can also become leptin resistant.

**Leptin resistance** occurs when the body no longer responds properly to leptin signals. Despite high leptin levels, the brain fails to recognize that the body has sufficient energy stores, which increases hunger and reduces energy expenditure. This condition is often associated with weight gain or inability to lose weight (no matter what diet and exercise program you're struggling to maintain) and can also disrupt normal metabolic functions.

Proper circadian rhythm has a massive influence on leptin levels and function. Leptin levels typically follow a daily cycle, peaking during the night and decreasing in the daytime. Disruption of the circadian rhythm, such as staying up late or being exposed to artificial light at night, can affect leptin production and signaling. This dysregulation can contribute to leptin resistance, creating metabolic issues and making it hard to maintain a normal body weight. Effective management of circadian rhythm is important for maintaining leptin sensitivity and supporting healthy metabolic function.

# Insulin Resistance

The next casualty of poor circadian rhythm is **insulin resistance**. **Insulin** is a hormone produced by the pancreas that plays a vital role in regulating blood sugar levels. It allows the glucose to be used to create cellular energy and helps the body store extra glucose in the liver as glycogen. This process ensures that blood sugar levels remain within a healthy range and offer up a steady supply of energy.

Insulin resistance occurs when cells in the body become less responsive to the effects of insulin. As a result, the pancreas produces more insulin to compensate, which can eventually lead to Type 2 diabetes. Factors like obesity, sedentary lifestyle, and genetic predisposition can contribute to the development of insulin resistance. Symptoms of insulin resistance include:

- Weight gain
- Increased hunger and thirst
- Frequent urination, headaches
- Darkening of the skin in folds and creases
- Vaginal and skin infections
- Slow-healing cuts and sores

The modern working woman is a prime target for insulin resistance. Sitting all day and eating high-fat, high-carbohydrate, highly processed meals can elevate blood glucose and insulin levels.

Research indicates that poor circadian rhythms can make insulin resistance worse. Irregular sleep patterns, shift work, and exposure to artificial light at night can disrupt the body's internal clock, leading to metabolic imbalances.

One study showed that night shift workers had higher levels of insulin resistance compared to day workers, partly due to circadian misalignment (4). Further research showed that people with irregular sleep schedules also had greater insulin resistance, *even if they were eating a healthy diet and engaging in regular exercise* (5).

Night shift workers are exposed to LED and blue light throughout the nighttime hours, which throws off their natural circadian rhythms and can cause major metabolic problems. This means that artificial light from screens and lightbulbs can actually contribute to perimenopausal weight gain by increasing insulin resistance.

# Insulin Resistance and Sleep

Insulin resistance not only impacts blood glucose levels but also has negative effects on sleep quality, leading to insomnia and fatigue. Several studies support this connection, showing a link between metabolic health and sleep.

One study found that people with higher levels of insulin resistance were more likely to experience poor sleep quality and shorter sleep duration (6). The dips and spikes in blood sugar and the hormonal imbalances associated with insulin resistance can affect the body's natural sleep-wake cycles. This can make it harder to get to sleep and to stay asleep.

Another study in *PLOS One* reported that people with insulin resistance often experience increased levels of inflammation and stress hormones like cortisol (7). Especially in the evening, high cortisol levels can disrupt the body's ability to initiate and maintain sleep.

Chronic sleep deprivation can worsen insulin resistance, creating a vicious cycle that perpetuates both weight and sleep issues. When you're not sleeping well, you often put on weight. And when you put on weight, you might sleep even more poorly. Getting outside at regular intervals from sunrise to sunset can help your body regulate both sleep and weight.

# Melatonin and Circadian Rhythm

Melatonin is another major player in circadian rhythm balance. Melatonin is a hormone primarily produced by the pineal gland in response to darkness and plays an important role in regulating sleep-wake cycles and circadian rhythms. Emerging research tells us that melatonin also impacts metabolic processes, including leptin regulation.

A study published in the *International Journal of Endocrinology* highlighted that when people with poor metabolic function were given a melatonin supplement, their leptin sensitivity was restored (8). The study showed that melatonin supplementation improved leptin signaling pathways, improving appetite regulation and reducing caloric intake. *When we get regular exposure to the sun and secrete normal amounts of melatonin, our bodies may spontaneously eat fewer calories.*

Research from *Sleep Medicine Reviews* showed that melatonin can help synchronize leptin secretion to align with the body's natural circadian rhythm and in turn, help to maintain metabolic health (9). When our circadian rhythms are off because we don't get enough natural sunlight during the day or we are regularly exposed to screens after dark, leptin is not produced appropriately. This can make us hungrier! And when we're hungry late at night, we're rarely choosing chicken breasts and broccoli. We're in the pantry, face-deep in tortilla chips or granola. *Getting regular exposure to daytime sunlight helps us produce normal levels of melatonin at the proper times and this in turn can regulate our appetite.*

A study in the *Journal of Pineal Research* showed that when clinically obese people were given melatonin supplementation at bedtime, they became more leptin-sensitive and could better discern when they were hungry and when they were full (10). *This study showed that melatonin not only decreases leptin levels at night, enhancing the body's energy balance during sleep, but also reduces the risk of metabolic disorders associated with elevated leptin levels.* If you're waking up hungry in the middle of the night, odds are your leptin levels are off. If this is a struggle for you, start working on getting regular daytime sunlight exposure as soon and as often as possible.

I don't recommend just going out and buying a melatonin supplement. Melatonin is a powerful hormone. It is possible to take too much melatonin, especially for children. My recommendation is to simply get outside at sunrise and sunset to give your brain the proper signals to make its own melatonin, naturally.

And remember: over-exercising, over-stressing, and over-dieting can significantly disrupt circadian rhythms, contributing to insulin resistance and leptin resistance. These disruptions in circadian rhythms can seriously mess with your hormones and can make you over-tired. The research is clear. *Stress messes with our appetite, weight, and sleep.* **The Overs** are not your friend when it comes to proper circadian rhythm and correct signaling of hormones like leptin and insulin.

Let's talk a little more about each one of **the Overs** so you can understand why I'm encouraging you to break free from your desire to constantly be and do more.

# Over-Exercising

Excessive exercise can lead to overproduction of cortisol. A study published in the *Journal of Sports Sciences* found that high-intensity exercise raised cortisol levels and disrupted the circadian rhythm (11). Another study in *Medicine & Science in Sports & Exercise* showed that disruption of circadian rhythm led to insulin resistance (12). When we push our bodies too hard with excessive exercise, our body responds by excreting high levels of cortisol. That's exactly what we're trying *not* to do.

**The purpose of Easy Perimenopause is to lower stress hormone levels.** And as the research shows, balanced cortisol levels lead to balanced insulin levels, which make it easier for us to keep our weight stable. It's funny how many of my clients stop going to Orangetheory, training for half marathons, and doing CrossFit and begin to slowly lose weight. When they were exercising excessively, their bodies just didn't feel "safe" enough to lose weight. Perimenopause is your pass to drop your gym membership and buy yourself a cute, brand-new pair of walking shoes.

## Over-Stressing

Chronic stress also affects circadian rhythms by consistently elevating cortisol levels. Research in the *Journal of Clinical Endocrinology & Metabolism* showed that lengthy periods of stress led to leptin resistance, which contributed to overeating and weight gain (13). We women already inherently know that we tend to overeat when we're stressed. But now you know that you're not just weak-willed or undisciplined.

When you're under a lot of stress for a long period of time, leptin can no longer send "I'm full!" signals to the brain. Your hormones are actually trying to help you. When the body senses that it is in danger due to elevated stress hormones, it wants to protect you by making sure you have plenty of calories to fight off whatever stressor is affecting you at that time. You can give your hormones a hand by learning how to manage your stress effectively.

Women in perimenopause are more susceptible to acquiring Type 2 diabetes. As estrogen levels decline, our bodies can no longer as effectively process glucose and we become more insulin resistant. To add insult to injury, elevated cortisol due to chronic stress disrupts insulin signaling pathways, as evidenced by a study in *Diabetes Care*. This elevated cortisol increases the risk of insulin resistance and Type 2 diabetes (14).

See how that cycle perpetuates itself? It's empowering to realize that you have control over your metabolic health. As you manage stress and eat a nourishing diet, you may decrease your chances of getting Type 2 diabetes.

# Over-Dieting

Speaking of diet, we need to address our collective love affair with unintended malnutrition. When we cut calories drastically or chronically, we deprive ourselves of necessary nutrients. The problems don't stop there. Now that you're familiar with how important a healthy circadian rhythm is to metabolic health, you're going to want to use all of the tools in your toolbox to dial in your circadian health. Chronically cutting calories will royally mess with exactly that.

The *American Journal of Clinical Nutrition* found that severe caloric restriction disrupted natural circadian patterns of both leptin and insulin (15). This disruption means big problems for glucose regulation, making us more leptin- and insulin-resistant. On top of that, the stress associated with extreme dieting can further elevate cortisol levels and compound these negative effects.

Remember, leptin resistance disrupts the body's ability to regulate hunger and energy expenditure. When the brain becomes less sensitive to leptin, it can't tell whether or not you're actually full. This leads to cravings for unhealthy foods and can also cause us to overeat, even if we don't actually need of more food.

Studies have demonstrated the connection between leptin resistance and weight gain. A landmark study published in *Cell Metabolism* found that higher levels of circulating leptin were associated with increased body fat in both rodents and humans (16).

Another study in the *Journal of Clinical Investigation* highlighted that people start to become leptin-resistant before they begin gaining significant weight, suggesting leptin resistance may be an early marker for obesity (17). This all might sound a bit complicated, but it's actually easy to understand when you see the flow, start to finish.

**Chronic stress/imbalanced circadian rhythm >
high cortisol > high insulin and leptin >
insulin and leptin resistance > weight gain**

If we work backwards with the objective of wanting to lose weight or keep a stable weight, the flow looks like this:

**Desire to lose weight >
restore insulin and leptin sensitivity >
reduce stress > lose weight**

# Planning your Optimal Circadian Day

Begin to plan your day to optimize your circadian rhythm. Get outside for five minutes around sunrise and look to the eastern horizon, being careful not to stare directly at the sun. View the sunrise. This allows broad-spectrum UVA and UVB sunlight to activate your pineal gland and allows the brain to tell the body to start producing normal amounts of cortisol—not too much, not too little.

Get outside for a few minutes at regular intervals throughout the day. I block off short breaks in between each client appointment so I can spend about five minutes in the sun, multiple times a day.

I have a wise and resourceful client named Summer who works eight hours a day in an office. Summer came up with a clever solution to her circadian rhythm problem. Every time she has to use the restroom, she exits her building and walks all the way around it before re-entering and heading to the bathroom. It takes her eight minutes, from start to finish, and she gets about five minutes of outside time multiple times a day. I love this!

If you have young children, take them outside often. If you work from home, take a meeting or two on your front porch or have Zoom "walking meetings." If you're homeschooling, do science class outside. If you're a caregiver, go for a stroll with your charge a few times a day. If you're in a car or stuck inside, open up the window—the healing UVA and UVB rays cant get through window glass. And just a note—even if it's rainy, snowy, or cloudy outside, the sun's rays are still able to send the correct hormone signals to your brain. Get outside, even in inclement weather. Your ancestors did!

Finally, check the weather app on your smartphone to determine when sunset will occur each day. Try to be outside for a few minutes right around this time, gazing toward the western horizon so your brain realizes the sun is setting and it's time to shut down cortisol production and start melatonin production.

I guarantee if you can spend this much time outside each day, you'll notice a positive difference in your cravings, stress levels, mood, and sleep.

# Circadian Rhythm Action Items

- **Spend five minutes outside at sunrise.** If possible, don't wear glasses or contacts during this time. If you're up before the sun, wear blue blockers inside until the sun rises and you can get outside. If you're up after sunrise, make sunlight the first thing you see—not your phone TV, or tablet.
- **Get outside for five minutes multiple times a day.** Ideally, this would be at 10 a.m., 12 p.m., 2 p.m., and 4 p.m. Just make it work for your schedule.
- **Spend five minutes outside** around sunset.
- **Try to spend as much or more time outside** as you do inside, especially on the weekends as your schedule permits.

CHAPTER 7:

# Supplements – Big Promises, Disappointing Results

As AN FDN practitioner, I'm trained to help clients interpret their functional lab tests. I love using data to help perimenopausal women develop an action plan for their frustrating hormonal and gut symptoms. After being left behind by the traditional medical community, many women come to someone like me for alternative care options. They don't just want a pill or medication.

Many of these women are also under the false impression that if they could just find the right supplement, their mood/energy/weight/libido/gut/hormones would be balanced. It's the social media trap—once your phone hears you say the word "hormone" or "perimenopause," your social media channels will start offering you a buffet of shiny and sexy supplements. Don't fall into that trap! *Supplements are just that—supplements to a healthy lifestyle, not fix all of our medical problems.* The dietary supplement industry is large and growing, with a global market size of $146.14 billion in 2023, and it's largely unregulated (1). It's very likely that the supplement you bought off of Instagram isn't as effective as it claims to be.

## Heather

"So, what should I take?" Heather asked. She had come to me with pretty severe gut issues, and we had just run one of my favorite functional labs—the GI Map (*you're going to learn more about all of my favorite lab tests later!*). Heather and I were sitting in a Zoom session, discussing her results. I could see the September afternoon sunlight streaming through her window, highlighting the distress on her pretty face. Heather had suffered from bloating and stomach pain for months. It was a good thing that we ran her GI Map, as she had multiple bacterial overgrowths in her gut, along with a poor number of good bacteria and a nasty strain of yeast called *Microsporidium*. Her immune function was low, and she had a stomach bacteria called *Helicobacter pylori* that made her stomach acid less acidic and more alkaline, so her digestive system couldn't break down her food properly.

Heather had been a victim of the system for some time. She had been experiencing gut issues for years. When she complained to her medical professionals, her symptoms were glossed over and she was essentially dismissed. My notes from our session read like this:

> *No matter how clean Heather eats, she is always bloated. She has IBS all of the time, and if she splurges, she is instantly sick. This has been going on for a long time, at least a few years. She is having severe stomach cramps. Her anxiety is high too.*

# Supplements are Just Supplements

When we find imbalances in gut tests, as we did in Heather's case, targeted supplements will be a key part of a rebalancing protocol. But as I stress to my clients, we might use pills and potions and powders as a short-term intervention for targeted support, but pills and potions and powders are not a long-term solution.

With Heather, we ended up using some digestive support and a powerful spore-based probiotic. These things helped. But more importantly, we changed the way that Heather viewed food. She began to remove foods that triggered her stomach symptoms, and she also focused on getting more dietary protein. She got back to me two years after making the changes we put into place for her.

"I also still don't eat dairy, soy, and gluten and still eat a load of meat too. That helps with my anxiety for sure!"

Note what she didn't say: *"I'm still taking five pills and three powders."* She was managing her frustrating gut symptoms all by herself, through diet, rest, and stress management. These are the long-term interventions that make a real difference in the lives of women with hormone, gut, mood, sleep, libido, and energy issues.

# Supplements Aren't Substitutes for a Healthy Lifestyle

I find it intriguing that so many people eat processed and packaged foods, drink endless amounts of coffee on an empty stomach, skip meals in favor of snacks, regularly drink alcohol, stay up late, and invite stress into their lives, and then think that a pill is going to solve the problems come from these life choices. This isn't a knock on anyone—it's just a normal part of Western culture, especially for driven, high-performing women.

One key misunderstanding is that *supplements aren't a substitute for a healthy lifestyle.* Many people mistakenly believe they can simply supplement their way out of a poor diet or stress-laden life. This approach is like putting a bandage on a broken limb; it may cover the issue temporarily, but it doesn't solve the underlying problem. As their name indicates, supplements are designed to *supplement*—to add to or enhance—not to serve as a substitute for the essentials: a balanced diet rich in protein, whole foods, and staying out of chronic fight-or-flight mode. *Supplements just cannot fix* the Overs. Our bodies are remarkably capable of balancing hormones when given the right support: food, exercise, and stress reduction.

## Supplements Are Largely Unregulated

There's another problem with supplements. In the USA, the supplement industry is largely unregulated. This means the quality and concentration of ingredients can vary widely, so that some products that may even do more harm than good. Additives like guar gum and magnesium stearate can cause digestive issues or other health problems for unsuspecting consumers.

I've seen women who buy every supplement Instagram throws at them and then wonder why their gut issues are getting worse (and their hormone issues aren't getting better!). Young girls on social media are particularly vulnerable to this trend. I can't tell you the number of times my seventeen-year-old daughter has sent me a TikTok with a shiny influencer promoting some pill or potion, asking me to buy her the fifty-dollar "miracle in a bottle." And I'll tell you what I tell her: *if you aren't getting enough protein, calories, sleep, or time each day in parasympathetic nervous system dominant mode, no amount of Irish sea moss will grow your hair out healthy and strong.*

A recent example of an unregulated supplement problem is the discovery of unapproved stimulants in several weight-loss supplements marketed for fitness, in which researchers identified compounds similar to ephedrine (a previously banned dangerous weight-loss ingredient) in products with no prior FDA review or listing of these ingredients on the label (2). This highlights the issue of potential adulteration in the supplement market without strict regulation.

I can guarantee you that your great-great-great-great grandmother did not have a supplement drawer. Or a supplement cabinet. Or a supplement room. She just ate whole and healthy food in sufficient quantities to get her macronutrients and her micronutrients. She didn't overthink her health, and she certainly didn't put much stock in a quick fix. And we shouldn't, either. It's a false bill of health feeding into the desire for rapid resolutions. No supplement can replicate the benefits of consuming ample protein and the necessary micro and macronutrients—nor can they combat the impacts of the stress hormone cortisol on the body.

# Supplements Should be Personalized

Each person's need for supplementation should be based on individual data derived from functional lab tests. This personalized approach ensures that supplements are used strategically and effectively, rather than as catch-all remedies.

With Heather, we implemented a few strategic, short-term supplements based on her gut test results. And we got results. But lo and behold, Heather recently reached out to me concerned about histamine issues:

*"I'm having histamine reactions to things. I itch after I eat most foods. Sometimes I'm fine; other times I'm not."*

I asked Heather what exactly she'd been eating, and she shared that she had recently added apple cider vinegar (ACV) and also ACV gummies to help with digestion. Cider vinegar is a fermented food, and fermented foods are associated with histamine responses in the body; anything aged or fermented can increase histamine levels in the blood. Since she had seen ACV advertised as a healthy supplement, Heather assumed it was safe and beneficial for her. But when she removed the vinegar, her itchy skin began to clear up.

## Supplements Are Often Unnecessary

If a supplement isn't making a noticeable difference, it may not be necessary. Your body is intelligent; if you're not experiencing benefits, it's time to reconsider your regimen. Don't take supplements without a *reason* to take supplements.

Supplements must be repositioned in our minds. They are not a cure-all, especially during the sensitive period of perimenopause. *Instead, they are a potential short-term aid when added to a well-balanced lifestyle.* Remember, food always has been and always should be our primary source of nutrition—not an afterthought next to a pile of pills. It's time to refocus on the basics of nutrition and mindfulness before leaning on the crutch of supplements. It's a less glamorous path, but certainly a more effective, sustainable, and healthier one, especially in the long run.

## Food-Based Supplements Can be Safer and More Effective Than Pills

Food-based supplements can be a beautiful addition to the perimenopause transition. I have three primary recipes I share with clients, and these recipes cover a wide range of hormone and gut-related imbalances. They're easy to make at home, and they end up being cheaper and more sustainable than a pill. I call them my **Core Hormone Recipes,** and they are designed to balance **the Overs**. These are food-based interventions to help manage the effects of previous over-dieting, overstressing, and overexercising.

## The Lemon Gut Shot

I start all of my clients off with the **Lemon Gut Shot** because nearly all of my girls have gut issues. Gas, bloating, slow gut motility, constipation, and even acid reflux benefit from the Lemon Gut Shot. If you experience diarrhea regularly, this won't be a food supplement you'll want to start off with, due to the quickening action of the lemon and the spices. But if you have any other gut or tummy problems, here's the recipe I want you to start with:

## The Lemon Gut Shot

**Ingredients:**

- 1 lemon, whole, with white pith
- 2 tsp ground ginger

- 1 tsp ground cinnamon
- 2 tsp ground turmeric
- 1 cup water

**Instructions:**

- Peel your lemon but leave as much of the white pith on as possible. Use a high-speed blender to thoroughly blend all ingredients, adding more water if you want to make it thinner. Store in a glass mason jar in the refrigerator. Shake well before serving each day. Drink 1 oz every morning on an empty stomach. If under the weather or constipated, drink up to four servings a day.
- This will keep for up to five days in the refrigerator. Feel free to substitute fresh ginger and turmeric for the ground powders.

Lemon, ginger, turmeric, and cinnamon are beneficial for various tummy issues. Lemon aids digestion, ginger reduces bloating, turmeric helps with gas and inflammation, and cinnamon can alleviate reflux and constipation. I usually have clients start with one shot glass of the Gut Shot on an empty stomach each morning. For clients with more severe pain, bloating, or gas, I'll encourage them to take a shot glass full before every meal until symptoms abate. Generally, relief is felt within a few days.

# The Adrenal Cocktail

The second Core Hormone Recipe is the **Adrenal Cocktail**. To be fair, I didn't create this recipe. It's been around the mineral wellness sphere for ages, and for good reason. Most women are woefully deficient in fight-or-flight-balancing minerals like sodium and potassium. Do you feel like you can never get enough salt? For a period of time, I added salt to my *coffee* because my body was crying out for increasing amounts of sodium to deal with fight-or-flight mode!

When I run the hair tissue mineral analysis (HTMA) on clients, I routinely see extremely low levels of sodium and potassium in the hair. The HTMA provides a three-month picture of mineral status in the body. Imagine being super low on potassium for months or years at a time. You'll have cravings, your thyroid hormone won't be able to get into the cells, and you'll have a hard time losing weight. This is a pattern I see routinely. And few people are talking about the need for potassium (except Marty Kendall.)

We need to focus on our minerals, and the Adrenal Cocktail is a highly effective way to balance minerals and get out of fight or-flight mode. Note that I didn't say it's a *tasty way* to get out of fight-or-flight mode—it's salty! And with good reason. You need the sodium and the trace minerals found in a high-quality salt to feel optimal in perimenopause. Here's the recipe:

## The Adrenal Cocktail

**Ingredients:**

- ½ cup orange juice, any brand, no sugar added
- ½ cup coconut water, any brand, no sugar added
- ¼ tsp pink Himalayan or Celtic salt
- 1 scoop collagen powder (Great Lakes is a good brand)
- ¼ tsp cream of tartar

**Instructions:**

- Mix all ingredients in a thermos or mason jar and screw the lid on tight. Shake vigorously until all ingredients are mixed well. Sip slowly over a few hours to get a steady supply of minerals throughout the day.
- Make an Adrenal Cocktail during times of extra stress, insomnia, or illness. If your stool gets loose after drinking this due to the sodium and potassium, simply cut back on your serving size or discontinue use for a few days.

Cream of tartar offers a significant source of potassium. Potassium acts like a balm, soothing an overtaxed nervous system. The orange juice is contains plenty of easily digested sugar and vitamin C—both helpful tools in adrenal health. Coconut water offers another source of bioavailable potassium. I find that a mix of coconut water and orange juice is less taxing on blood sugar. A gray Celtic or pink Himalayan sea salt will replace sodium and trace minerals that bring the body back into balance quite quickly. I encourage you to add a scoop of collagen powder (I like Great Lakes or Vital Proteins) to your Adrenal Cocktail to get further blood sugar-balancing effects. This is also a great way to sneak in more protein.

Make a full serving of the Adrenal Cocktail and put it in a thermos. Sip on it throughout the day, when you feel stressed, anxious, or low in energy. Make a second serving and leave it by your bedside table. If you wake up in the middle of the night, a few sips should get you back to dreamland, quickly.

# Cramp-Free Energy Bites

The third Core Hormone Recipe is the **Cramp-Free Energy Bites**. Not only are these absolutely delicious, but they will help you balance out the hormonal roller coaster of perimenopause. Flax seed functions as a phytoestrogen and can have one of two effects: if you're high in estrogen, it will block the estrogen cell receptor site from attracting the potentially more toxic estradiol. If you're low in estrogen, it will fit the estrogen cell receptor site and function as a weak estrogen. The combination of oats and flax helps decrease cramps and breast pain that tend to show up with a perimenopausal period.

The recipe makes twenty servings, and I recommend you eat one yummy serving a day. The honey, chocolate, and peanut butter are my gift to your perimenopausal sweet tooth. Kids and husbands can enjoy these, too. The Bites won't have any negative effects on their hormones. In fact, my college-aged son and my two young teenage boys routinely request that I whip up a batch of these. And my daughter's volleyball friends love it when there is a fresh supply of the Bites in the Woodward fridge.

## Cramp-Free Energy Bites

**Ingredients:**

- 1 cup old fashioned oats
- ⅔ cup shredded coconut (sweetened or unsweetened)
- 2/3 cup creamy peanut butter
- ½ cup ground flaxseed
- 1 cup high-quality milk or dark chocolate chips
- ⅔ cup honey

- 1 tbsp chia seeds
- 1 tsp vanilla extract
- Optionally, 2 scoops collagen powder (I like Great Lakes Quick Dissolve collagen peptides)

**Instructions:**

- Mix all ingredients in a large mixing bowl until thoroughly combined. Roll the mixture into 1-inch balls and store in an airtight container in the refrigerator or freezer. If the dough is not sticky enough, add 1 tbsp of peanut butter at a time until it sticks well. If it is too sticky, add in 2 tbsp oats at a time until it is a perfect consistency.

Since my family goes through these so quickly, I make a triple batch each week. You might want to do the same!

# Final Thoughts on Supplements

- Supplements are there to help, not to take over. Focus on real food first.
- Think of supplements as a guest appearance in your life, not the main character.
- The supplement world is a wild west. Make sure you know what you're dealing with.
- Your body and your doctor should be your go-to guides—not some flashy Instagram ad.
- When in doubt, eat real food. It's what your body craves and recognizes.
- Start with food-based supplements like the Lemon Gut Shot, the Adrenal Cocktail, and the Cramp-Free Energy Bites.

CHAPTER 8:

# Is It My Thyroid?

KAT'S SYMPTOMS WERE making her feel crazy, and she was worried she was going to snap. A vibrant, petite blonde mom of three, she spent her minimal free time serving in the prayer group at school and volunteering in her children's classrooms. Although she always looked cheerful and put together, the stress of working, parenting, and caring for a young daughter with Type 1 diabetes was clearly taking a toll on her health.

Kat was desperate to figure out why her normally 120-pound body had ballooned up to 160 pounds. No amount of diet or exercise seemed to affect the weight gain. She had been to her family doctor several times and had recently visited an endocrinologist. One year prior, Kat had been diagnosed with hypothyroidism, and she had been taking levothyroxine ever since. Even with the medication, Kat was exhausted and had to nap every single day. Her doctors ran blood work and declared, *"Your thyroid numbers look normal!"*

Discouraged, she came to me with the desire to lose weight and get her energy back. Kat already exercised, ate well, and did her best to manage her stress. Before adjusting anything in her life, I encouraged her to ask her doctor for an expanded thyroid panel.

*"My doctor thought I was crazy but ran the tests. After the tests were run, it occurred to you that the levothyroxine was*

121

*not working and you recommended that I ask my doctor to switch me to natural desiccated thyroid. In three months, twenty pounds came off and my energy was back.*"

Kat and I also implemented a nourishing diet with plenty of protein and minerals. We focused on getting outside, walking, and taking Epsom salt baths. We talked about prayer and journaling, and Kat began to take a few targeted supplements.

Kat messaged me recently after I put a post about thyroid health on my social media:

*"I'm laughing at the 'Did you know thyroid blood work can look normal?' You're telling my story; you solved my two-year mystery and saved me from insanity!"*

## What Is the Thyroid?

The thyroid gland is a butterfly-shaped gland located in the front of the neck, right below the Adam's apple. It produces hormones that regulate many important bodily functions, including:

- **Metabolism**: Thyroid hormones control how quickly the body uses calories from food.
- **Growth and development**: These hormones are essential for proper growth and development in children and adolescents.
- **Heart rate and blood pressure**: Thyroid hormones affect the heart rate and blood pressure.
- **Mood and cognitive function**: They also play a role in mental and neurological health.
- **Body temperature**: Thyroid hormones help regulate body temperature.

The thyroid gland produces two main hormones: **thyroxine** (T4), the inactive form of the hormone; and **triiodothyronine** (T3), the active form of the hormone.

## The Thyroid Is Not an Isolated Organ

The thyroid is a complicated gland, especially for women. It's unwise to think of your thyroid as an isolated organ. If you're struggling with your weight or energy levels, it's not just your thyroid. By this point in the book, you understand that as fearfully and wonderfully made as women's bodies are, they are complex creations that are rightly sensitive to disturbances in diet, sleep, and stress.

## The HPT Axis

Let me introduce you to the hypothalamus-pituitary-thyroid (HPT) axis. We have already discussed the hypothalamus-pituitary-adrenal (HPA) axis as it relates to stress management and the central nervous system. But the hypothalamus and pituitary glands drive the function of many organs in the body other than the adrenal glands. The **HPT axis** is a network that regulates metabolism, energy levels, and overall hormonal balance. This finely-tuned balance begins when the hypothalamus produces thyrotropin-releasing hormone (TRH), which stimulates the pituitary gland to secrete thyroid-stimulating hormone (TSH). TSH then drives the thyroid gland to produce T4 and T3, which have major effects on almost every physiological process.

The relationship between these three glands ensures a delicate equilibrium within the body's hormonal systems. Let's stop right here for a moment and take note that *most doctors will only run a TSH test when looking for markers of thyroid dysfunction.* You now know that TSH is a hypothalamic hormone. **TSH doesn't actually measure thyroid hormone itself.** For perimenopausal women, the HPT axis is especially significant. Our thyroid hormones play a central role in managing symptoms and maintaining health during this time. Thyroid hormones influence numerous functions, from reproductive health to bone density and cardiac function. An imbalance in this axis can worsen certain symptoms associated with the perimenopause transition.

# Inflammation and the Thyroid

As you've already learned, decades of dysfunction in the body—and overexposure to **the Overs**—can create high levels of systemic inflammation. Inflammation is harmful to the thyroid system in a few key ways. First, it lowers the production and regulation of important thyroid hormones, as demonstrated by research in which a single inflammatory trigger reduced thyroid hormone levels for several days. This indicates that while thyroid medications might replace some hormones, *they don't tackle the underlying issue of inflammation's impacts on hormone production and regulation.*

Secondly, inflammation can reduce the quantity and function of the receptors that thyroid hormones need to work on in the body. It's akin to someone lowering the volume on their hearing aid; no matter how loud you speak, they can't hear you. Lastly, inflammation hampers the body's ability to convert inactive T4 into active T3. This is problematic because most thyroid medications only provide T4, which won't help someone who can't effectively convert T4 to T3 due to inflammation.

Taking natural or bioidentical hormones, which include both T4 and T3, may be more beneficial for those affected by this issue. This was the case for Kat. When she transitioned from a T4-only medication to a T4/T3 combination in the form of natural desiccated thyroid hormone, her body responded much better. *Of course, medication is something you would need to discuss with your doctor. I'm not a doctor; I'm simply an educator.*

## TSH Isn't Enough

Measuring TSH alone is a poor method for assessing thyroid function because it doesn't provide a complete picture of the hypothalamus-pituitary-thyroid (HPT) axis's performance or the body's overall hormonal balance. TSH levels can fall within normal ranges even when there are significant issues with thyroid hormone production or action within the body. Without measuring the thyroid hormones T3 and T4, which directly affect metabolism, energy, and physiological processes, it's challenging to accurately diagnose or manage conditions related to thyroid dysfunction. This approach overlooks the nuanced interplay between TSH and the thyroid hormones, potentially missing subclinical or early-stage thyroid issues.

TSH tells only part of the story—how stressed your brain and body are. TSH tells the thyroid to output more T4. The liver must then convert that T4 into T3 for thyroid hormone to actually be used by the cells. To make this conversion, you must have adequate levels of dietary iodine and selenium. It's estimated that up to 45% of people worldwide are deficient in iodine, and one billion of us are selenium deficient (1, 2).

Interestingly enough, deficiency of both iodine and selenium is correlated with greater rates of anxiety and depression

(3). If, as a typical perimenopausal woman, you're addicted to **the Overs** and you have been undernourished for years or decades, you're likely deficient in these vital nutrients and your thyroid function is likely compromised.

## Why Thyroid Hormone Replacement Therapy Might Not Work

During prolonged periods of stress, the presence of cortisol in the bloodstream actually prevents conversion of T4 into T3 and instead uses T4 to create a hormone known as **reverse T3** (4). Reverse T3 is made from T4 when the body is out of balance.

Why is this a potential problem? Reverse T3 can bind to a cell in the same way T3 does, except reverse T3 can mimic all of the symptoms of low thyroid hormone. When your body creates more reverse T3 than free T3, you may feel exhausted, chubby, and cold.

Reverse T3 fits onto the same cell receptor site as free T3 and can essentially block thyroid hormone from doing its job. *This is why medications like Synthroid (levothyroxine) may feel like they are not working for you, as T4-only medications can be converted into reverse T3 as well as free T3.* Inflammation is a major factor in the creation of reverse T3 as opposed to free T3 (5). Lack of quality sleep has also been shown to drive up T3 levels (6).

The use of natural desiccated thyroid (NDT) or T3-only medications (liothyronine) won't be any more helpful for your symptoms if you are still addicted to **the Overs**. Thyroid meds won't fix your thyroid issue—what you have is a lifestyle issue. That's not to say that thyroid medication cannot be beneficial, because it certainly can! But if you feel like your meds aren't working, ask yourself if you're doing the right things when it comes to nutrition, exercise, circadian rhythm, and stress management.

Thyroid hormone conversion can be a bit confusing, so let me take you back to my junior high years, when I cut my own bangs, sewed my own flannel shirts, and played the string bass in the Tevis Junior High Orchestra.

## The Thyroid Symphony

Imagine your body as a grand symphony orchestra, with each instrument playing a crucial role in creating beautiful music. In this orchestra, TSH is the thoughtful conductor, ensuring that everything runs smoothly. With a wave of the conductor's baton, TSH signals to the thyroid gland to produce T4, the primary hormone, much like the violins starting the melody.

Now, T4 is versatile, but it's not quite ready to shine as the star soloist. It needs to transform into T3, the active hormone, which is like the lead violinist stepping forward for a breathtaking solo. This transformation is facilitated by various enzymes—our tireless stagehands—working diligently behind the scenes.

However, sometimes things don't go as planned. Instead of converting into T3, some of the T4 can turn into reverse T3 (rT3), a bit like an unexpected musical note that doesn't fit the harmony and disrupts the performance. This is where the environment and tools come into play. For the orchestra to perform at its best, the stagehands need the right conditions—adequate nutrition, minimal stress, and optimal health. When these factors are in place, the transformation from T4 to T3 happens seamlessly, and the symphony plays in perfect harmony.

The body knows that when you are stressed, sleeping poorly, and eating an inadequate diet, it must conserve all of its available energy. It will hold onto every calorie you eat and slow down metabolic functions. Thyroid medications cannot replace a nourishing diet, deep sleep, and proper rest. If the body is stuck in fight-or-flight mode, all the thyroid medication in the world will not help you lose weight and gain energy.

## The Thyroid-Gut Connection

The health of your digestive system also plays an important role in the conversion of T4 to T3, which takes place in the gut. Problems like dysbiosis (an imbalance between beneficial and pathogenic gut bacteria), inflammatory bowel disease, and high intestinal permeability or "leaky gut" can impair the body's production of active T3 hormone. As 20% of thyroid hormone conversion happens in the gut, caring well for your digestive tract is especially important (7). In the presence of dysbiosis (which I routinely see in my clients after running a test like the GI Map), thyroid hormone conversion can become increasingly weak, and perimenopausal symptoms like weight gain, body temperature issues, and heavier periods can become more and more common.

# The Autoimmune Connection

TPO (thyroid peroxidase) and TG (thyroglobulin) antibodies are indicators of autoimmune thyroid conditions like Hashimoto's thyroiditis and Graves' disease, where the body's immune system mistakenly attacks the thyroid gland. Testing for these antibodies is important for perimenopausal women because hormonal changes during this period can increase or trigger thyroid dysfunction, impacting overall health.

# Ask Your Doctor For These Labs

It's a good idea to get regular thyroid lab testing in perimenopause. If you are asking your doctor for thyroid labs, make sure to request that he or she test:

- Free T4
- Total T3
- Reverse T3
- TSH
- TPO antibodies
- TG antibodies

If your doctor is only testing TSH (or even T4) while neglecting to look at total T3 and reverse T3 levels, you may be told that your labs are normal even when your body is unable to properly utilize thyroid hormone.

## Normal Thyroid Hormone Levels

| Lab Marker | Reference Range |
|---|---|
| TSH (Thyroid-stimulating hormone) | 0.5-5.0 IU/mL |
| Free T4 | 0.7–1.9 ng/dL |
| Total T4 | 5.0-12.0 µg/dL |
| Total T3 | 80-220 ng/dL |
| Reverse T3 | 10-24 ng/dL |
| TPO (thyroid peroxidase) antibodies | < 35 IU/mL |
| TG (thyroglobulin) antibodies | < 0.9 IU/mL |

Table 3: Normal Thyroid Marker Ranges (8)

# Minerals and the Thyroid

To add another layer to the thyroid discussion, our mineral levels are major players in the body's ability to utilize thyroid hormones. I routinely run hair tissue mineral analyses on my clients, and about 90% of the time, I find elevated levels of calcium and very low levels of potassium in the hair tissue. When calcium is being leached from the bones into the soft tissue, it can begin to accumulate around the cell membranes. Because calcium is a hard and brittle mineral, this can cause the cell walls to become impermeable. This prevents thyroid hormone from getting into the cells to do its work. When potassium levels are low, the sodium/potassium pump becomes less efficient.

There is a cause-and-effect relationship at play here. Those with low thyroid function tend to suffer from low electrolyte status, including sodium, chloride, and potassium. As we have already seen, most of us aren't getting enough potassium in our diets. Increasing dietary potassium can improve mineral balance and bring thyroid function back online. Minerals are like the spark plugs of the body, providing the raw materials for energy creation (9).

## My Secret At-Home Thyroid Tests

There are at-home indicators of robust thyroid function as well. In the book *Hypothyroidism: The Unsuspected Illness* (1976), thyroid researcher Dr. Broda Barnes claimed that hypothyroidism was much more prevalent than previously believed (10). Barnes argued that low thyroid function was the player behind many of the chronic health issues are common among Westerners, including obesity, heart disease, diabetes, hormone dysfunction, and even cancer.

He developed the "Barnes Basal Temperature Test," a diagnostic tool for assessing thyroid function. The procedure involves taking one's temperature in the armpit right after waking up for a total of ten minutes. It's recommended that perimenopausal women conduct the test on the second and third day of their menstrual cycle to ensure accuracy.

According to Barnes, a basal temperature below 97.8 degrees Fahrenheit (or 36.6 degrees Celsius) is a strong indication of hypothyroidism, particularly when accompanied by symptoms associated with the condition. This simple test provided an accessible means of identifying potential hypothyroidism in people and is my first secret at-home thyroid test. You can check your own thyroid function by taking your temperature every morning before you get out of bed. Use any thermometer you have. If you're using a digital thermometer, take your temperature three times and record the average.

The second secret at-home thyroid test involves monitoring your resting heart rate (RHR). Heart rate decreases in the presence of low thyroid function (11). Those with hypothyroidism often have heart rates of 10 to 20 beats per minute (BPM) slower than usual.

A normal heart rate is 60 to 90 BPM. You can use an inexpensive monitor to determine your RHR. If you're not an elite athlete and your RHR routinely falls between 40 to 70 BPM, it is likely that you have a degree of hypothyroidism (12).

The heart muscle requires thyroid hormone as well as calcium and potassium for proper contraction and relaxation. When the thyroid functions properly, the heart beats at a steady pace, about 60 BPM. When the thyroid is low functioning, the pulse will drop. Interestingly, I have seen that when my clients increase their potassium and sodium intakes, their heart rates tend to normalize.

# Cortisol, Stress, and Thyroid Hormone

Dr. Barnes approached treatment of hypothyroidism by initially prescribing a low dosage of thyroid hormone to his patients, gradually increasing it on a monthly basis until the patient's symptoms improved and their basal body temperature reached a range between 97.8°F and 98.2°F. As thyroid function normalized, the resting heart rate also returned to normal. He advised that the dosage should not exceed three grams (or 180 mcg) of desiccated thyroid. Continuing this optimal dosage for life was recommended for many patients. However, there were cases in which the dosage could be reduced gradually. Barnes predominantly used a particular brand of desiccated thyroid extract, Armour Thyroid, believing that it was more effective than synthetic thyroid hormone.

# It's the Adrenals
## *(It's Always the Adrenals!)*

Barnes grew to believe that a large portion of his patients with hypothyroidism also suffered from undiagnosed adrenal insufficiency—cortisol issues! So, he often prescribed prednisone, a synthetic corticosteroid, especially to those whose systolic blood pressure was under 100.

The more recent literature supports Barnes' theory that cortisol and thyroid hormone are inextricably linked. Few practitioners these days address both the adrenals (cortisol) and the thyroid at the same time. Cortisol regulates the transport mechanism that gets thyroid hormone into the cell (13). If cortisol happens to be too low—which I also see regularly in my practice—it also means that thyroid hormone cannot be effective. It is imperative to normalize cortisol levels before attempting to "fix" the thyroid. *Thyroid health starts with adrenal health.* Impaired adrenal activity is likely the reason your thyroid medication has stopped working or never worked in the first place.

*To further educate yourself on thyroid health, visit the excellent patient education website* Stop the Thyroid Madness *(https://stopthethyroidmadness.com). See www.jenniferwood-wardnutrition.com/resources for more information.*

In my own practice, I find that as adrenal health becomes more robust, thyroid function also begins to normalize. When perimenopausal women remove the shackles of **the Overs** and begin to eat enough food, get enough sleep, and manage stress appropriately, all hormones begin to come back into balance.

I have never seen thyroid hormone alone "fix" a woman with weight, mood, or temperature dysregulation. *Both naturally produced and supplemental thyroid hormones can only work if the nervous system is properly balanced and regulated.* The published literature supports this; hypothyroidism is associated with greater sympathetic nervous system (fight-or-flight) activity and less parasympathetic nervous system (rest and digest) activity (14). Other studies have shown a strong link between the adrenals and the thyroid (15). When adrenal function is compromised, overall metabolic health suffers, which means the slowing of metabolism can start with decreased thyroid function.

# Dr. Ray Peat And Pro-Metabolic Nutrition

Another excellent source for thyroid education is researcher and biologist Dr. Ray Peat. Dr. Peat's work spans metabolic health, aging, and environmental stressors, among other topics. He has published numerous articles and books that challenge conventional medical wisdom. Most of his writings focus on thyroid function, progesterone, and the role of dietary nutrients in maintaining optimal health. Dr. Peat passed away in 2022, but many of his books can be found online for free. His website is also a treasure trove of information on hormonal health, metabolism, and the thyroid.

The thyroid gland was one of Dr. Peat's obsessions. He fathered the concept of *pro-metabolic nutrition*, which refers to eating in a way that increases metabolism (read: helps you lose weight). I personally love much of Dr. Peat's work. However, he is an advocate of a fairly high-carbohydrate diet. I have found that while plenty of carbohydrates can certainly be quite healing for a body that has been a victim of t**he Overs** for a long time, excess carbohydrates can also be a surefire way to put on even more perimenopausal weight. So, feel free to start getting "Peat-y." But keep in mind that as a perimenopausal woman, you need fewer carbohydrates than a twenty-year-old woman or even a forty-year-old man.

Pro-metabolic nutrition consists of nutrient-dense foods that promote cellular energy production and lower cortisol levels. On a pro-metabolic diet, all macronutrient groups have relatively equal weight. Peat recommended prioritizing easily digestible carbohydrates from fruits, roots, and dairy. He encouraged regular consumption of high-quality proteins from sources like milk, cheese, eggs, and gelatin. He was an advocate for removing toxic seed oils from the diet, preferring saturated fats over polyunsaturated fats, which he believed could slow metabolic function.

Dr. Peat knew the thyroid gland was crucial for maintaining overall health. He wrote, "The thyroid hormone is crucial, not just for metabolism, but for every tissue in the body. Ensuring adequate levels of thyroid hormone is essential for maintaining health and vitality" (15).

How do we maintain adequate levels of thyroid hormone? By refusing to continue being victims of **the Overs**.

Stop over-dieting. Include a modest amount of healthy carbohydrates in your diet and eat plenty of protein. Good news—there's an entire suggested meal plan provided for you at the end of this book! And the meal plan is quite pro-metabolic. Listen to Dr. Peat on the subject: *"By prioritizing the consumption of easily digestible carbohydrates and high-quality proteins, individuals can create a supportive environment for their thyroid to function effectively"* (15). According to Peat, easily digestible carbohydrates include fruits and carrots. Both of these are included in your suggested meal plan. In fact, you'll be introduced to Dr. Peat's **Raw Carrot Salad** as an afternoon snack.

## Peat's Raw Carrot Salad

Peat advocated for the consumption of his Raw Carrot Salad as a simple and powerful dietary tool for better hormone health. Carrots are rich in dietary fiber and promote gut health, helping the body get rid of excess estrogen and toxins. Peat emphasized that eating the carrots raw helps to preserve the vital nutrients and enzymes that support digestive health and metabolic function. Carrots also provide a natural source of antioxidants that combat oxidative stress and further contribute to hormonal balance and thyroid function. The suggested meal plan in the back of the book includes regular consumption of the Raw Carrot Salad.

But remember: *"It's not just about what you eat, but how you manage stress. Reducing stress is vital for optimal thyroid activity and overall hormonal balance"* (15). So said Peat. Even a seemingly perfect diet can't fix a body stuck in fight-or-flight mode. In fact, trying to pursue a perfect diet can *keep* you in fight-or-flight mode. This is because there is no perfect diet. That should be a freeing sentence!

Rather than focusing on trying to be the best at dieting, seek to look at your nutrition through the lens of true nourishment. In fact, the word *diet* comes from the Greek word *diaita*, meaning *way of life*. Our diets should reflect the way we live. And we should live to nourish ourselves, not try to starve ourselves skinny and silly.

As part of this plan, you'll be adding in protein, collagen, and plenty of raw carrots. But you'll also be getting outside, observing the sunrise, taking Epsom salt baths, getting to bed on time, practicing breath work, and moving your body in a stress-free manner. All of these factors work together to bring your thyroid function back into balance.

Kat's restored thyroid health is allowing her to enjoy life again. We saw each other recently at a Halloween-themed birthday party, though I barely recognized her. Not only has she kept off her forty-pound weight loss, but she showed up to the party dressed as the titular character from *Beetlejuice*. We hung out on the dance floor for hours, enjoying the music, the great company, and the thyroid-fueled energy that allowed both of us to boogie the night away.

## Thyroid Action Items

- **Use a tracking app** like Cronometer to record your potassium intake throughout the day. Aim to get at least 5,000 mg of potassium if you struggle with thyroid symptoms. Include foods like avocados, bananas, and white potatoes to increase your potassium. Use the recipe for Potassium Broth for an easy way to get 1,000 mg of potassium at a time.

- **Get the right labs from your doctor:** TSH, free T4, free T3, and reverse T3. If your doctor won't run the labs, you can order them for yourself.
- Consider running an HTMA to look at pertinent minerals, including your calcium and potassium levels.
- **Normalize adrenal function** before attempting to use thyroid medication. If cortisol levels are too high or too low, natural and/or synthetic thyroid medication likely won't be effective against symptoms like fatigue, weight gain, and low body temperature. Consider checking your cortisol levels.
- **Add a scoop or two of collagen powder** to your morning beverage or in a smoothie, as Dr. Peat suggests.
- **Cut out inflammatory seed oils** like canola, soy, corn, sunflower, and safflower oil.
- **Commit to your stress-managing habits**: baths, walking, outside time, breath work, and sleep.

For more information, see **www.jenniferwoodwardnutrition.com/resources.**

CHAPTER 9:

# Case Studies

IN THIS CHAPTER, I want to give you a closer look at some of my clients. I have been working with perimenopausal women for the better part of a decade, and I've seen a lot of the same patterns. As you read their stories, assess who you identify the most with. You'll be able to use their stories and successes as a blueprint for your own rebalancing program.

## *Whitney*

Whitney is one of the original CrossFitters. She was doing AMRAPs before CrossFit was cool. As a busy mom of two, she cut out the gym middleman and built a "box" in her garage so she and her fire captain husband could work out together.

Whitney counted macros diligently for years and maintained her fit, willowy figure. Tall with glossy brunette hair, she has the Instagram-perfect image that most women want.

But as with most things in life, the image didn't tell the whole story. One night I was sitting in my backyard, watching my husband grill us dinner on the barbecue. I got the following text from Whitney:

> *"Can I set up an appointment with you? My body is failing me."*
> *"Of course," I texted back. "What's going on?"*

She replied:

*"In the fall of 2019, I was having episodes where I would just suddenly wake up with no energy, really dizzy. In 2022 I had long COVID, so I just took a long time to get my energy back. In the last six to eight months, there's been probably a week a month where I feel like I have energy. I've also had a really sensitive stomach. I'm always bloated.*

*"I feel like it's been hard to lose weight. I don't know if I've gained weight, but I just feel like my lower stomach area is 'poochy.' It feels like I've gained weight, even though it's not showing on the scale, and when I've done different things to try to lean out, I can't.*

*"I'm doing all the things like high protein—I eat 1,900 to 2,000 calories a day. I switched over from CrossFit a couple of years ago, so I just do weightlifting. And I try to walk. I know I'm definitely not getting 10,000 steps. Especially with working full-time, sitting at a desk.*

*"It's getting to the point where I feel like I can't function like this anymore. I went to the doctor and he just said you're just getting older and you're a mom and you're working and of course you're tired… but it's more than just being tired. And that's what I need your help with."*

I highlight Whitney because I hear a variation of this same story *almost every single day.* Low energy, no results from working out, lower belly pooch, and being dismissed by doctors—these symptoms hallmarks of perimenopause. I could not have written her case study better myself.

## *Whitney's DUTCH*

Instead of guessing why Whitney was experiencing the issues she was struggling with, we went right to work and ran the Dried Urine Test for Comprehensive Hormones (DUTCH).

Visit www.jenniferwoodwardnutrition.com/resources for more information on this and other tests.

The DUTCH is an at-home dried urine test taken over a period of about twelve hours. The test collects five urine samples to look at estrogen, progesterone, testosterone, DHEA, melatonin, cortisol, adrenaline, B vitamin markers, and more.

Whitney's DUTCH showed estrogen dominance, meaning her estrogen levels were higher than her progesterone levels. This can make it impossible to lose weight, even while working out and eating well. She also had extremely high cortisol levels, with a cortisol spike at night. This prevented her from losing belly fat and robbed her of energy, as her body was in fight-or-flight mode all of the time. Her DUTCH also showed that she was spilling indican into her urine. This suggested that she was not breaking down her dietary protein effectively, which likely accounted for some of her diarrhea and bloating.

Low dopamine levels on the DUTCH indicated imbalance in her circadian rhythm, as a lack of vitamin D from sunshine is directly associated with lower dopamine levels. We also ran a functional blood chemistry panel on Whitney and found low vitamin D levels (35.5 ng/mL), which further suggested her circadian rhythms were off. Because Whitney worked a desk job inside during normal daylight hours, she was not getting the proper sun and UVA/UVA exposure she needed to make vitamin D and dopamine.

## Whitney's Blood Work

On a hunch, we also tested Whitney's Epstein-Barr virus (EBV) antibodies and they were extremely high (>600/ EBV CA, IgG; 592 EBV nuclear antigen Ab, IgG). Extreme fatigue is one of the hallmarks of a chronic reactivated viral infection like EBV. You can ask your doctor to test for this panel if you are struggling with chronic unexplained fatigue. Then you can take steps to support yourself.

*Dr. Kasia Kines is a leading expert on chronic EBV infection and has an excellent website on the subject (https://kasiakines.com). Visit www.jenniferwoodwardnutrition.com/resources for more information.*

## Whitney's Plan

Whitney's customized plan included cutting down on heavy workouts, removing raw fruits and vegetables to decrease bloating, removing her whey-based protein powder to curb diarrhea, getting plenty of animal protein with each meal, walking outside in the sun for about four to five miles a day as she was able, and including a spore-based probiotic and a few herbs to manage her hormonal symptoms. We added vitamin D and K2 to raise her low vitamin D, but I also recommended that she try to spend thirty to sixty minutes in the sun each day. We also removed gluten from her diet, which immediately firmed up her stool and cut down on bloating.

## Whitney's Results After Three Months

Three months into her program, Whitney reported the following:

- Sleep has been great
- Energy has been great
- Able to work out again and not "crash"
- Getting daily walks in
- Digestion has been great, with no IBS in months!
- Feeling so good

By running the labs and curating an individualized protocol, Whitney was able to feel like her old self fairly quickly. Even without the labs, following the advice in Easy Perimenopause should also help you feel like yourself again ASAP.

Now that you've heard Whitney's journey, let's take a closer look at Elisa's story.

## *Elisa*

You've already met Elisa—she's one of the inspirations for this book. I love talking about her story because she made such an incredible transformation by doing the exact things I'm sharing with you in this book. Elisa's intake form was one of the most overwhelming I've ever read. Here was the list of her symptoms:

- "Low blood pressure"
- "Adrenal fatigue with a diagnosis of Addison's Disease"
- "Intolerance to dietary protein"
- "Gallbladder issues (not tolerating much fat or nuts), nausea, pain, etc."
- "GERD"
- "Lots of digestion issues"
- "Reflux from mild to severe in times of stress"
- "Blood sugar imbalance"
- "30 pounds overweight"
- "Perimenopause—erratic periods, tender breasts"
- "Long history of endometriosis & severe ovarian cysts"
- "Exhausted all the time, but I can't sleep"
- "TMJ, neck, and jaw issues"
- "Working out has resulted in crashing for days as well as weight gain (not muscle)"
- "Regular intense headaches"

- "Very little appetite"
- "Often nauseated from smells (especially in the AM)"
- "No libido"
- "Hormonal migraines"
- "Hiatal hernia"
- "Spider veins/varicose veins. With not much pressure on my legs or feet at all, I will feel the sting and boom, there's a new one."
- "I 'crash' often."

*Elisa had experienced these concerns for a long time*, some for twenty or more years. Other symptoms, like her gallbladder issues, insomnia, and being unable to tolerate much physical exertion without crashing, had been bothering her for the past four years.

Elisa is a Total Transformation private client, so we ran all of the labs on her; we tested her hormones, thyroid, immune system, food intolerances, gut, brain, and blood chemistry.

## Elisa's Lab Test Results

Notable finds from the labs included the following:

- Very low vitamin D
- Low serotonin, dopamine, GABA, and 5-HTP *(when all of these brain neurotransmitters are low, one may feel depressed and anxious)*
- Extremely low good gut bacteria
- High anti-gliadin antibodies *(indicating a strong sensitivity to gluten)*
- Multiple food intolerances, including to cruciferous vegetables, caffeine, MSG, soy, garlic, and wheat
- Estrogen dominance with tanked progesterone levels

- Nonexistent testosterone
- Elevated cortisol
- Low B vitamins
- Mineral imbalances

Elisa was no stranger to eating well and caring for herself and her family, as her two young daughters also had health issues that mandated a special diet. She easily made the food changes requested, removing her trigger foods and slowly increasing her protein. As we re-established the proper beneficial gut bacteria, she was able to tolerate more protein. This crucial step allowed her body to begin the hard work of rebuilding itself from decades of malnourishment.

## Getting Out Of Fight Or Flight Mode

We cut out all exercise except walks, and Elisa began spending more time outside. We prioritized increasing dietary minerals like potassium and sodium so her nervous system started to calm down and she began sleeping better. She began asking for more help with things around the house and at work. Her week-long headache spells began to decrease and eventually completely subside.

## Elisa's Results

After a few months of working hard on getting enough food, we went into a weight loss phase and Elisa dropped from 171 to 145 pounds. During this cut, we worked hard to preserve her nervous system function so that she was still sleeping, pooping, and feeling energized even in her weight loss phase. She was even able to take a ski vacation that would have previously been impossible with all of her health issues. Elisa just recently messaged me and let me know that she is now at 125 pounds, a year after starting her Easy Perimenopause journey. Amazing!

At the end of our time together, Elisa wrote, "I am stronger (physically and mentally). I am calmer (inside and out). I can handle all the things with so much more grace and confidence because I can trust my body again! My body is forgiving me for over twenty-five years of being abused and mistreated."

While the labs were important in figuring out the specific imbalances in Elisa's body, the principles remain the same. We prioritized proper nourishment and digestion, circadian rhythm, stress management, and sleep. When she was stronger, we worked on exercise and fat loss. You too can do these things by following the principles laid out for you in this book. Commit to fighting **the Overs** and prioritize your nourishment so your body can calm down and rebalance itself.

## Should I Go on Hormone Replacement Therapy (HRT)?

Estrogen replacement therapy (ERT) alone has been associated with an increased risk of endometrial cancer. This risk arises because estrogen stimulates the lining of the uterus, which can lead to excessive growth and potential malignancy if not counteracted by progesterone. According to a study published in the Journal of the National Cancer Institute, women using unopposed estrogen therapy showed a significantly higher incidence of endometrial cancer compared to those using combined estrogen-progesterone therapy (1). Another study highlighted in the Women's Health Initiative found that **adding progesterone to estrogen therapy mitigates this cancer risk by inducing regular shedding of the en-**

**dometrial lining** (2). A further NIH study confirmed these findings, emphasizing the importance of combined hormone therapy for the safety of long-term users (3). *In short, HRT can be extremely beneficial and very safe for women when prescribed correctly by a knowledgeable physician and when used in conjunction with a healthy lifestyle plan like the one suggested in this book.*

Western women often make hormone dysfunction worse through their lifestyle choices, such as excessive dieting, high-intensity exercise while fasting, and high consumption of coffee and alcohol—all compounded by chronic stress and insufficient sleep. You now know these as **the Overs**. These practices can lead to hormonal imbalances, particularly during the critical transition period of perimenopause. A comprehensive review published in the American Journal of Obstetrics and Gynecology demonstrated that these stressors negatively affect adrenal and thyroid function, which in turn disrupts estrogen and progesterone balance (4). Addressing these lifestyle factors holistically can contribute to a more balanced hormonal transition and reduce the need for medical interventions.

However, some women benefit from going on HRT. If you're ready to talk to your doctor about getting on estrogen, make sure you are informed. Bring a copy of this book, and make sure you discuss adding protective progesterone to your hormone stack. And if you are on HRT and you don't feel any difference, make sure that you're working on dialing in your nutrition, exercise, stress management, sleep, and lifestyle first. Once these things are dialed in, it's likely that you will start to feel more positive effects from your HRT.

**Hormones and Optimal Blood Levels** (35-55 Year Old Cycling Perimenopausal Women)

| Hormone | Possible Benefits | Possible Risks | Optimal Blood Levels |
|---|---|---|---|
| Estradiol | • Supports bone health<br>• Maintains heart health<br>• Enhances mood | • Increased risk of breast cancer<br>• Blood clots<br>• Stroke | 30-400 pg/mL |
| Progesterone | • Regulates menstrual cycle<br>• Reduces PMS symptoms<br>• Supports pregnancy | • Weight gain<br>• Fatigue<br>• Mood swings | **Follicular phase**: 0.1–0.7 ng/mL<br><br>**Luteal phase**: 2–25 ng/m |
| DHEA | • Boosts energy levels<br>• Supports immune function<br>• Improves libido | • Acne<br>• Mood changes<br>• Hair loss | 30-280 µg/dL |
| Testosterone | • Increases muscle mass<br>• Enhances mood<br>• Improves cognitive function | • Hair growth (facial/body)<br>• Deepening of voice<br>• Mood swings | 15-70 ng/dL |

Table 4: Optimal Hormone Blood Levels for Cycling Perimenopausal Females

## CHAPTER 10

# Daily Meal Plan

Commit to this plan for three months and see how you feel. Live simply. Eat simply. Channel your great-great-great grandmother. Eat locally and in season like she did. Skip the gym and walk outside a lot like she did. Use herbs and whole foods as supplements like she did. Sync your body and brain to the rhythms of nature like she did. These are the steps to an Easy Perimenopause. And you can do this, too.

Here's a full 14-day meal plan. I've made this plan as easy as possible so that you can prepare a healthy meal in under thirty minutes. This plan gives you about 1,800 calories a day. Some of you may need more than that, and some of you may need less. But try to commit to this general plan for 28 days before you start going around changing everything, so you can give it a fair shake. Simply find the recipes you like and repeat them every 14 days.

## Substitutions

It's easy to substitute. If you don't like a particular animal protein (like beef), you can use another animal protein (like chicken or fish). Substitute any vegetable for another vegetable, any fruit for another fruit, and any nut or legume for another nut or legume. If you don't care for a certain meal, simply double the recipe for a meal you do like and eat it twice that week. This plan is not meant to be rigidly prescriptive, but to act as a helpful guide.

## Portion Sizes

If you need more food, increase your meal sizes. If you need less food, decrease your meal sizes or skip a snack. If you are sleeping well, pooping well, feeling energized, and enjoying a balanced mood, you've likely hit your nutrition sweet spot.

## Cooking for Your Family

Your family will like these meals, too. Mine do. My clients' families do. Just multiply the portion sizes by the number of people in your family. I have four kids. I need *simplicity*. My recipes are tasty, filling, and nourishing and use minimal ingredients. Even your high school or college kid could follow this plan.

*P.S. If you're having a Cramp-Free Energy Bite each day, just omit the suggested sweet evening snack.*

# Easy Perimenopause Suggested 14-Day Meal Plan

## Day 1

*P.S. Prep your Chia Seed Pudding for dessert.*

## BREAKFAST: Scrambled Eggs with Spinach and Avocado

### Ingredients:

- 3 large eggs
- 1 cup spinach, chopped
- 1/2 avocado, sliced
- 1 tbsp olive oil

### Instructions:

- Heat olive oil in a pan over medium heat.
- Add spinach and sauté until wilted.
- Whisk eggs and pour them into the pan.
- Cook, stirring frequently, until scrambled.
- Serve with sliced avocado on the side.

**Total:** 457 cals, 20g protein, 40g fat

## SNACK #1: Apple Slices with Almond Butter

**Ingredients:**

- 1 medium apple, sliced
- 2 tbsp almond butter

**Total:** 295 cals, 6g protein, 18g fat

## LUNCH: Gluten-Free Roll-Up

**Ingredients:**

- 5 oz roast turkey lunch meat
- 1 cup arugula
- 1/2 cup sliced apples
- 2 tsp honey mustard
- 1 tbsp shaved parmesan cheese
- 2 gluten-free tortillas

**Instructions:**

- Brush 1 tsp honey mustard onto each tortilla.
- Layer meat, arugula, apples, and parmesan.
- Roll up and eat.

## SNACK #2: Ray Peat's Raw Carrot Salad

**Ingredients:**

- 1 large carrot, grated
- 1 tbsp coconut oil, melted
- 1/2 lemon, juiced

**Instructions:**

- Mix grated carrot with coconut oil and lemon juice.

**Total:** 156 cals, 1g protein, 14g fat

# DINNER: Roasted Filet with Veggies

**Ingredients:**

- 6 oz steak filet
- 1 cup broccoli florets
- 1 cup sweet potatoes, diced
- 1 tbsp olive oil

**Instructions:**

- Preheat oven to 400°F (200°C).
- Place filet on a baking sheet and season as desired.
- Toss vegetables with olive oil and spread around steak.
- Bake for 20–25 minutes, or until steak is slightly pink in the middle and potatoes are cooked through.

**Total:** 557 cals, 43g protein, 21g fat

# EVENING SNACK: Chocolate Chia Pudding

**Ingredients:**

- 2 tbsp chia seeds
- 1 cup almond milk
- 1 tbsp cocoa powder
- 1 tsp honey

**Instructions:**

- Mix all ingredients together in a bowl.
- Refrigerate for at least 2 hours or overnight.

**Total:** 183 cals, 6g protein, 11.5g fat

# Day 2

*Peel and freeze a banana for dessert tonight.*

## BREAKFAST: Greek Yogurt Parfait

**Ingredients:**

- 1.5 cups plain nonfat Greek yogurt
- 1/2 cup mixed berries
- 1/4 cup granola

**Instructions:**

- Layer yogurt, berries, and granola in a bowl or glass.

**Total:** 285 cals, 28g protein, 8g fat

## SNACK #1: Ray Peat's Raw Carrot Salad

(see recipe from Day 1)

## LUNCH: Apple Tuna Salad Wraps

**Ingredients:**

- 5 oz canned tuna
- 1 tbsp capers
- ½ cup finely diced celery
- 4 cups finely diced apple
- 1 tbsp organic mayonnaise
- 4 large lettuce leaves
- Salt and pepper to taste

**Instructions:**

- Mix drained tuna in a bowl with capers, celery, apple, and mayo.
- Spoon onto lettuce leaves and roll up.

**Total:** 315 cals, 29g protein, 5g fat

## SNACK #2: Almonds and Blueberries

**Ingredients:**

- 1/4 cup almonds
- 1/2 cup blueberries

**Total:** 242 cals, 6g protein, 18g fat

## DINNER: Grilled Shrimp and Veggies

**Ingredients:**

- 6 oz shrimp
- 1 cup zucchini, sliced
- 1/2 cup cherry tomatoes
- 1 tbsp olive oil

**Instructions:**

- Toss shrimp and veggies in olive oil and season as desired.
- Grill until shrimp is opaque and vegetables are tender.

**Total:** 295 cals, 35g protein, 16g fat

## EVENING SNACK: Banana "Nice Cream"

**Ingredients:**

- 1 frozen banana
- 1 tbsp almond butter

**Instructions:**

- Blend frozen banana until smooth.
- Swirl in almond butter.

**Total:** 205 cals, 4g protein, 9g fat

# Day 3

## BREAKFAST: Avocado Toast with Eggs

**Ingredients:**

- 3 eggs, poached
- 1/2 avocado, mashed
- 2 slices gluten-free bread

**Instructions:**

- Poach eggs.
- Spread mashed avocado on toasted gluten-free bread.
- Top with poached eggs.

**Total:** 460 cals, 24g protein, 27g fat

## SNACK #1: Cucumber Slices with Hummus

**Ingredients:**

- 1 cup cucumber slices
- 1/4 cup hummus

**Total:** 116 cals, 3g protein, 6g fat

## LUNCH: Quinoa and Black Bean Salad

**Ingredients:**

- 1 cup cooked quinoa
- 1/2 cup black beans, rinsed
- 1/4 cup red onion, chopped
- 1/2 cup cherry tomatoes, halved
- 2 tbsp olive oil & lime dressing

**Instructions:**

- Combine quinoa, black beans, red onion, and cherry tomatoes.

- Drizzle with olive oil & lime dressing and toss to coat.

> **Total:** 605 cals, 15g protein, 32g fat

# SNACK #2: Ray Peat's Raw Carrot Salad

(see recipe from Day 1)

# DINNER: Turkey Meatballs with Zoodles

**Ingredients:**

- 6 oz ground turkey
- 1 egg
- ⅛ tsp garlic salt
- 1 cup zucchini noodles
- 1/2 cup marinara sauce

**Instructions:**

- Heat oven to 400 degrees.
- Form ground turkey, egg, and garlic salt into 1-inch meatballs and bake for 20-25 minutes or until cooked through.
- Serve meatballs over zucchini noodles with marinara sauce.

> **Total:** 250 cals, 25g protein, 10g fat

## **EVENING SNACK:** Coconut Yogurt with Berries

### Ingredients:

- 1/2 cup coconut yogurt
- 1/2 cup mixed berries

### Instructions:

- Mix coconut yogurt with berries.

**Total:** 110 cals, 1g protein, 6g fat

# Day 4

## BREAKFAST: Smoothie Bowl

**Ingredients:**

- 1 cup almond milk
- 1 cup frozen berries
- 1 banana
- 1 tbsp chia seeds
- 1 tbsp almond butter
- 1 scoop Whole Feast
  Protein Powder
  (or similar)

**Instructions:**

- Blend almond milk, berries, protein powder, and banana until smooth.
- Top with chia seeds and almond butter.

**Total:** 365 cals, 8g protein, 15.5g fat

## SNACK #1: Hard-Boiled Eggs

**Ingredients:**

- 2 eggs

**Instructions:**

- Boil eggs for 10–12 minutes and peel.

**Total:** 140 cals, 12g protein, 10g fat

## **LUNCH:** Chicken and Vegetable Stir-Fry

**Ingredients:**

- 6 oz chicken breast, sliced
- 1 cup broccoli florets
- 1/2 cup bell pepper, sliced
- 1/4 cup carrots, sliced
- 2 tbsp coconut aminos

**Instructions:**

- Cook chicken in a pan until browned. Add salt and pepper to taste.
- Add vegetables and stir-fry until tender.
- Drizzle with coconut aminos.

**Total:** 257 cals, 35g protein, 4g fat

## **SNACK #2:** Ray Peat's Raw Carrot Salad

(see recipe from Day 1)

## **DINNER:** Beef and Vegetable Skewers

**Ingredients:**

- 4 oz beef sirloin, cubed
- 1/2 cup bell pepper, cubed
- 1/2 cup zucchini, cubed
- 1 cup white mushrooms, whole
- 1 tbsp olive oil

**Instructions:**

- Thread beef and vegetables onto skewers.
- Brush with olive oil and grill until cooked.

**Total:** 425 cals, 27g protein, 32g fat

# **EVENING SNACK:** Dark Chocolate Almonds

**Ingredients:**

- 1 oz dark chocolate
- 10 almonds

**Total:** 240 cals, 4g protein, 18g fat

# Day 5

## BREAKFAST: Veggie Omelete

**Ingredients:**

- 3 large eggs
- 1/4 cup bell pepper, diced
- 1/4 cup onion, diced
- 1/4 cup spinach, chopped
- 1 tbsp butter

**Instructions:**

- Heat butter in a pan over medium heat.
- Sauté bell pepper and onion until soft.
- Add spinach and cook until wilted.
- Whisk eggs and pour into pan.
- Cook until eggs are set.

**Total:** 363 cals, 19g protein, 29g fat

## SNACK #1: Celery with Almond Butter

**Ingredients:**

- 4 celery sticks
- 2 tbsp almond butter

**Total:** 215 cals, 7g protein, 18g fat

## LUNCH: Savory Tuna Salad Lettuce Wraps

**Ingredients:**

- 1 can tuna, drained
- 1/4 cup diced celery
- 1/4 cup diced red onion
- 2 tbsp mayo
- 4 large lettuce leaves

**Instructions:**

- Mix tuna, celery, red onion, and mayo.
- Spoon into lettuce leaves.

**Total:** 392 cals, 33g protein, 23g fat

## SNACK #2: Ray Peat's Raw Carrot Salad (see recipe from Day 1)

## DINNER: Baked Cod with Veggies

**Ingredients:**

- 6 oz cod filet
- 1/2 cup cherry tomatoes, halved
- 1/2 cup zucchini slices
- 1/4 cup red onion slices

**Instructions:**

- Preheat oven to 375°F.
- Place cod filet on a baking dish and top with cherry tomatoes, zucchini slices, and red onion.
- Bake for 15–20 minutes, until cod is cooked through.

**Total:** 190 cals, 34g protein, 1g fat

*P.S. Prep your Chia Seed Pudding for breakfast.*

# Day 6

## BREAKFAST: Chia Seed Pudding with Mango

**Ingredients:**

- 2 tbsp chia seeds
- 1 cup almond milk
- 1/2 cup diced mango
- 1 tsp honey

**Instructions:**

- Mix chia seeds, almond milk, and honey in a jar.
- Refrigerate for at least 2 hours or overnight.
- Top with diced mango before serving.

**Total:** 320 cals, 8g protein, 10g fat

## SNACK #1: Ray Peat's Raw Carrot Salad

(see recipe from Day 1)

## LUNCH: Cobb Salad

**Ingredients:**

- 4 oz shredded rotisserie chicken
- 1 tbsp precooked diced bacon
- 2 hardboiled eggs, halved
- ¼ avocado, sliced
- 3 cups diced romaine lettuce
- 2 tbsp organic ranch dressing

**Instructions:**

- Mix all ingredients together in a large bowl and toss well.

---

**Total:** 480 cals, 35g protein, 28g fat

---

## SNACK #2: Mixed Nuts

**Ingredients:**

- 1/4 cup mixed nuts (almonds, walnuts, cashews)

---

**Total:** 200 cals, 6g protein, 18g fat

---

## DINNER: Zucchini Noodles with Pesto Chicken

**Ingredients:**

- 4 oz grilled chicken breast
- 1 large zucchini, spiralized
- 2 tbsp pesto sauce (gluten-free)
- 1 tbsp pine nuts

**Instructions:**

- Spiralize zucchini to make noodles.
- Toss zucchini noodles with pesto sauce.
- Top with sliced grilled chicken and pine nuts.

---

**Total:** 400 cals, 38g protein, 20g fat

---

# EVENING SNACK: Berry Smoothie

### Ingredients:

- 1/2 cup mixed berries
- 1/2 banana
- 1 cup almond milk
- 1 tbsp chia seeds

### Instructions:

- Blend all ingredients until smooth.

**Total:** 300 cals, 8g protein, 12g fat

# Day 7

*P.S. Prep your Frozen Banana Bites for dessert.*

## BREAKFAST: Avocado Toast on Gluten-Free Bread

**Ingredients:**

- 2 slices gluten-free bread (I like Udi's or Base Culture)
- 4 oz turkey lunchmeat
- 1/2 avocado, mashed
- 1/4 cup cherry tomatoes, halved
- Salt and pepper to taste

**Instructions:**

- Toast gluten-free bread.
- Spread mashed avocado on toast.
- Top with cherry tomatoes, salt, and pepper.

**Total:** 450 cals, 26g protein, 23g fat

## SNACK #1: Ray Peat's Raw Carrot Salad

(see recipe from Day 1)

## LUNCH: Mexican Bowl

**Ingredients:**

- 1 cup instant brown rice
- ½ cup canned black beans, drained
- 6 oz rotisserie chicken, shredded
- 8 olives, sliced
- 1 tsp pumpkin seeds
- ⅓ cup salsa of choice
- 2 cups iceberg lettuce, shredded

**Instructions:**

- Mix all ingredients in a bowl and serve.

**Total:** 480 cals, 32g protein, 12g fat

## SNACK #2: Celery Sticks with Peanut Butter

**Ingredients:**

- 2 celery stalks, cut into sticks
- 2 tbsp peanut butter

**Instructions:**

- Dip celery sticks in peanut butter.

**Total:** 200 cals, 7g protein, 16g fat

## DINNER: Beef and Vegetable Skewers

**Ingredients:**

- 4 oz lean beef, cubed
- 1/2 bell pepper, cubed
- 1/2 zucchini, sliced
- 1/4 cup red onion, cubed
- 1 tbsp olive oil
- Salt and pepper to taste

**Instructions:**

- Preheat grill to medium-high heat.
- Thread beef, bell pepper, zucchini, and red onion onto skewers.
- Brush with olive oil and season with salt and pepper.
- Grill for 10–12 minutes, turning occasionally.

**Total:** 400 cals, 38g protein, 20g fat

# SNACK #2: Chocolate Banana Bites

## Ingredients:

- 1 banana, sliced
- 1 tbsp dark chocolate chips (dairy-free), melted

## Instructions:

- Drizzle melted dark chocolate over banana slices.
- Freeze for 30 minutes before serving.

**Total:** 300 cals, 4g protein

# Day 8

## BREAKFAST: Greek Yogurt Parfait

**Ingredients:**

- 1 cup plain Greek yogurt
- 1/2 cup mixed berries
- 1 tbsp chia seeds
- 1 tbsp honey
- 1/4 cup gluten-free granola

**Instructions:**

- In a bowl, layer Greek yogurt, mixed berries, chia seeds, and honey.
- Top with gluten-free granola.

**Total:** 300 cals, 20g protein, 10g fat

## SNACK #1: Apple Slices with Almond Butter

**Ingredients:**

- 1 medium apple
- 2 tbsp almond butter

**Total:** 200 cals, 4g protein, 16g fat

# LUNCH: Mediterranean Bowl

## Ingredients:

- 4 oz grilled chicken breast
- 2 cups mixed greens
- 1/4 cup cherry tomatoes
- 1/2 cup cucumber, diced
- 1 tbsp feta cheese
- 4 kalamata olives, sliced
- 1 tbsp lemon juice
- 1 tbsp olive oil

## Instructions:

- Mix all ingredients in a large bowl.

**Total:** 400 cals, 35g protein, 24g fat

# SNACK #2: Cottage Cheese with Pineapple

## Ingredients:

- 1 1/2 cups cottage cheese
- 1/2 cup pineapple chunks

## Instructions:

- Combine cottage cheese and pineapple chunks in a bowl.

**Total:** 150 cals, 20g protein, 5g fat

# DINNER: Roasted Steak Tips with Butternut Squash and Grapes

### Ingredients:

- 5 oz steak tips
- 1 cup butternut squash, cubed
- 1/2 cup red grapes, off the vine
- 1 tbsp olive oil
- 1 tbsp honey
- 1 tsp thyme
- Salt and pepper to taste

### Instructions:

- Preheat oven to 400°F (200°C).
- Place steak tips on a parchment-lined baking sheet and season with salt and pepper.
- Toss squash and grapes with olive oil, honey, thyme, salt, and pepper, and place around steak.
- Bake for 15–20 minutes until steak is cooked through and squash and grapes are tender.

**Total:** 450 cals, 28g protein, 22g fat

# EVENING SNACK: Dark Chocolate and Strawberries

### Ingredients:

- 1 oz dark chocolate (70% cocoa or higher)
- 1/2 cup strawberries

**Total:** 150 cals, 1g protein, 9g fat

# Day 9

*P.S. Prep your Chia Seed Pudding for later tonight.*

## BREAKFAST: Protein Smoothie

**Ingredients:**

- 1 cup almond milk
- 1 scoop Whole Feast Protein Powder (or similar)
- 1 small banana
- 1 tbsp almond butter
- 1 tbsp chia seeds

**Instructions:**

- Blend all ingredients until smooth.

**Total:** 350 cals, 25g protein, 12g fat

## SNACK #1: Carrot Sticks with Hummus

**Ingredients:**

- 1 cup carrot sticks
- 1/4 cup hummus

**Total:** 150 cals, 4g protein, 8g fat

## **LUNCH:** Quinoa and Black Bean Salad

**Ingredients:**

- 1/2 cup cooked quinoa
- ½ cup precooked rotisserie chicken, shredded
- 1/2 cup black beans
- 1/4 cup corn kernels
- 1/4 cup red bell pepper, diced
- 1/4 cup avocado, diced
- ½ tbsp lime juice
- 1 tsp olive oil
- Garlic salt and pepper to taste

**Instructions:**

- Mix all ingredients in a large bowl.
- Whisk lime, olive oil, garlic salt, and pepper together and toss with salad.

**Total:** 500 cals, 38g protein, 18g fat

## **SNACK #2:** Greek Yogurt with Blueberries

**Ingredients:**

- 1 cup plain Greek yogurt
- 1/2 cup blueberries

**Instructions:**

- Combine Greek yogurt and blueberries in a bowl.

**Total:** 150 cals, 15g protein, 5g fat

# DINNER: Green Tortilla Chili [makes 12 servings]

*My family likes to eat this with tortilla chips and sour cream.*

### Ingredients:

- 1 lb precooked rotisserie chicken, shredded
- 1 can jalapenos, diced
- 1 light beer (alcohol cooked off)
- 1 tbsp olive oil
- 1 cup frozen or fresh diced onions
- 2 (16 oz) jars of green salsa (I like Herdez or similar)
- 1 (40 oz) can of pinto beans, rinsed and drained
- 2 (32 oz) containers of organic chicken stock
- 1 tbsp cumin
- 2 tsp salt
- 1/2 cup cilantro, leaves only

### Instructions:

- In a large soup pot, heat olive oil.
- Add onions, jalapenos, and cumin, stirring slowly until onions are soft and translucent, about 5 minutes.
- Add beer and let alcohol cook off for about 5 minutes.
- Add chicken, beans, salsa, and chicken stock.
- Let simmer for 30 minutes.
- Top with cilantro and serve.

**Total per serving:** 350 cals, 26g protein, 22g fat

## **EVENING SNACK:** Chia Seed Pudding

### Ingredients:

- 1/4 cup chia seeds
- 1 cup almond milk
- 1 tbsp maple syrup
- 1/4 tsp vanilla extract

### Instructions:

- Mix chia seeds, almond milk, maple syrup, and vanilla extract in a bowl.
- Refrigerate overnight.

**Total:** 200 cals, 6g protein, 13g fat

# Day 10

*P.S. Prep Frozen Yogurt Bark for dessert.*

## BREAKFAST: Avocado Toast with Eggs [see recipe from Day 3]

## SNACK #1: Cucumber Slices with Guacamole

### Ingredients:

- 1 cup cucumber slices
- 1/4 cup pre-pared guacamole

### Instructions:

- Serve cucumber slices with guacamole.

---

**Total:** 150 cals, 2g protein, 12g fat

---

## LUNCH: Chicken and Veggie Stir-Fry

### Ingredients:

- 4 oz chicken breast, sliced
- 1 cup mixed vegetables (bell peppers, broccoli, snap peas)
- 1 tbsp olive oil
- 2 tbsp gluten-free soy sauce alternative (like coconut aminos)

**Instructions:**

- Heat olive oil in a pan and sauté chicken until cooked.
- Add mixed vegetables and stir-fry until tender.
- Drizzle with a gluten-free soy sauce alternative.

Total: 400 cals, 35g protein, 20g fat

## SNACK #2: Almonds and Dark Chocolate

**Ingredients:**

- 1/4 cup raw almonds
- 1 oz dark chocolate

Total: 200 cals, 6g protein, 18g fat

## DINNER: Peanut Shrimp and Noodles

**Ingredients:**

- 5 oz shrimp, peeled and deveined
- 1 tbsp jarred minced ginger
- ½ tsp ginger powder
- 1 cup brown rice spaghetti, cooked
- ½ cup sugar snap peas
- ½ cup shredded carrots
- 2 tbsp prepared peanut sauce

**Instructions:**

- Sauté garlic and ginger in olive oil until fragrant.
- Add shrimp and cook until pink.

- Cook brown rice pasta as directed.
- Toss shrimp, pasta, vegetables, and peanut sauce.

**Total:** 350 cals, 29g protein, 8g fat

# SNACK #3: Frozen Yogurt Bark

**Ingredients:**

- 1 cup Greek yogurt
- 1/4 cup mixed berries
- 1 tbsp honey
- 1/4 cup chopped nuts

**Instructions:**

- Spread Greek yogurt on a baking sheet lined with parchment paper.
- Top with mixed berries, honey, and chopped nuts.
- Freeze until firm, then break into pieces.

**Total:** 200 cals, 10g protein, 8g fat

# Day 11

## BREAKFAST: Berry Protein Smoothie Bowl

**Ingredients:**

- 1 cup almond milk
- 1 scoop whey protein powder
- 1 cup frozen mixed berries
- 1 tbsp chia seeds
- 1 tbsp almond butter

**Instructions:**

- Blend almond milk, protein powder, and frozen berries until smooth.
- Pour into a bowl and top with chia seeds and almond butter.

**Total:** 350 cals, 25g protein, 12g fat

## SNACK #1: Celery Sticks with Peanut Butter

**Ingredients:**

- 1 cup celery sticks
- 2 tbsp peanut butter

**Total:** 200 cals, 8g protein, 16g fat

# LUNCH: Lemony Chicken Grain Bowl

**Ingredients:**

- 4 oz precooked rotisserie chicken, shredded
- ½ cup instant brown rice
- ½ cup canned lentils
- 1 tbsp hummus
- ½ tbsp lemon juice
- 1/2 cup shredded carrots
- ½ cup diced romaine lettuce

**Instructions:**

- Toss all ingredients in a large bowl.

**Total:** 350 cals, 25g protein, 20g fat

# SNACK #2: Greek Yogurt with Honey and Walnuts

**Ingredients:**

- 1 cup plain Greek yogurt
- 1 tbsp honey
- 2 tbsp chopped walnuts

**Instructions:**

- Combine Greek yogurt, honey, and chopped walnuts in a bowl.

**Total:** 200 cals, 15g protein, 10g fat

# **DINNER:** Baked Cod with Cauliflower

**Ingredients:**

- 4 oz cod filet
- 1 cup cauliflower
- 1 small sweet potato, diced
- 1 tbsp olive oil
- Salt and pepper to taste

**Instructions:**

- Preheat oven to 375°F (190°C).
- Place cod on a baking sheet and season with salt and pepper.
- Toss cauliflower and sweet potato with olive oil, salt, and pepper, and place around cod.
- Bake for 15–20 minutes until cod is cooked through and cauliflower is tender.

**Total:** 350 cals, 30g protein, 15g fat

# **EVENING SNACK:** Banana Almond Ice Cream

**Ingredients:**

- 2 frozen bananas
- 1 tbsp almond butter

**Instructions:**

- Blend frozen bananas and almond butter until smooth and creamy.

**Total:** 200 cals, 4g protein, 8g fat

*P.S. Prep Overnight Oats for tomorrow.*

# Day 12

## BREAKFAST: Overnight Oats

**Ingredients:**

- 1/2 cup gluten-free oats
- 1 cup almond milk
- 1 tbsp chia seeds
- 1 tbsp almond butter
- 1/2 cup mixed berries
- 1 cup Whole Feast Protein Powder (or similar)

**Instructions:**

- Combine oats, almond milk, chia seeds, and almond butter in a jar.
- Refrigerate overnight.
- Top with mixed berries in the morning.

**Total:** 350 cals, 15g protein, 15g fat

## SNACK #1: Bell Pepper Slices with Hummus

**Ingredients:**

- 1 cup bell pepper slices
- 1/4 cup hummus

**Total:** 150 cals, 4g protein, 8g fat

## LUNCH: Tuna Salad

### Ingredients:

- 1 can tuna in water (drained)
- 1/4 cup diced celery
- 1/4 cup diced red onion
- 1 tbsp olive oil mayo
- 2 cups mixed greens

### Instructions:

- Mix tuna, celery, red onion, and mayo in a bowl.
- Serve over mixed greens.

Total: 400 cals, 35g protein, 15g fat

## SNACK #2: Greek Yogurt with Raspberries

### Ingredients:

- 1 cup plain Greek yogurt
- 1/2 cup raspberries

### Instructions:

- Combine Greek yogurt and raspberries in a bowl.

Total: 150 cals, 15g protein, 5g fat

# DINNER: Taco Bowl

## Ingredients:

- 5 oz cooked ground beef
- 2 tsp taco seasoning
- ½ cup canned black beans, drained
- ½ cup instant brown rice
- 2 tbsp prepared salsa
- ½ ripe avocado, diced
- ½ cup mixed diced bell pepper (red, yellow, green)

## Instructions:

- Sauté chicken breast with taco seasoning until cooked through.
- In a large bowl, toss meat, beans, rice, salsa, avocado, and bell pepper.

**Total:** 500 cals, 28g protein, 25g fat

# EVENING SNACK: Chocolate Avocado Mousse

## Ingredients:

- 1 ripe avocado
- 2 tbsp cocoa powder
- 1 tbsp honey
- 1 tsp vanilla extract

## Instructions:

- Blend all ingredients until smooth.

**Total:** 200 cals, 3g protein, 15g fat

## Day 13

## BREAKFAST: Egg and Veggie Scramble

**Ingredients:**

- 3 eggs
- 1/4 cup diced bell peppers
- 1/4 cup diced onions
- 1/4 cup spinach
- 1 tbsp olive oil
- Salt and pepper to taste

**Instructions:**

- Sauté bell peppers and onions in olive oil until tender.
- Add spinach and cook until wilted.
- Add eggs and scramble until cooked.
- Season with salt and pepper.

**Total:** 370 cals, 27g protein, 27g fat

## SNACK #1: Apple Slices with Almond Butter

**Ingredients:**

- 1 medium apple, sliced
- 2 tbsp almond butter

**Total:** 200 cals, 4g protein, 16g fat

# **LUNCH:** Quinoa and Chickpea Salad

**Ingredients:**

- 1/2 cup cooked quinoa
- ½ cup shredded pre-cooked rotisserie chicken
- 1/2 cup chickpeas
- 1/4 cup diced cucumber
- 1/4 cup cherry tomatoes
- 2 tbsp olive oil and lemon juice dressing

**Instructions:**

- Mix all ingredients in a large bowl.
- Drizzle with olive oil and lemon juice dressing.

**Total:** 500 cals, 38g protein, 28g fat

# **SNACK #2:** Greek Yogurt with Honey and Almonds

**Ingredients:**

- 1 cup plain Greek yogurt (can sub plant yogurt)
- 1 tbsp honey
- 2 tbsp sliced almonds

**Instructions:**

- Combine Greek yogurt, honey, and sliced almonds in a bowl.

**Total:** 200 cals, 15g protein, 10g fat

# **DINNER:** Chicken Thighs With Brussels Sprouts and Potatoes

## Ingredients:

- 2 medium-sized chicken thighs, bone-in and skin on
- 1 tbsp butter
- 1 cup Brussels sprouts, quartered
- 1 small white potato, diced
- ½ small onion, thinly sliced
- 1 tbsp olive oil
- 2 cloves garlic, minced
- 1 tsp seasoned salt

## Instructions:

- Preheat oven to 400 degrees.
- Heat butter in an oven-safe skillet until sizzling. Use a spatula to cover the pan in butter.

- Sprinkle ¼ tsp seasoned salt over each skin side of chicken.
- Toss sprouts, potato, garlic, onion in olive oil and remaining ½ tsp seasoned salt.
- Place chicken skin down in skillet. Cook for 3 minutes.
- Add Brussels sprouts, potato, garlic, and onion to the same skillet. Sauté, turning often.
- Turn chicken over and cook for another 3 minutes.
- Transfer to oven and cook at 400 degrees for 18–22 minutes, or until chicken is cooked through and vegetables are tender.

**Total:** 490 cals, 31g protein, 18g fat

# Day 14

*P.S. Prep Chia Seed Pudding for dessert.*

## **BREAKFAST:** Quinoa Porridge with Berries

### Ingredients:

- 1/2 cup quinoa
- 1 cup almond milk
- 1/2 cup mixed berries
- 1 tbsp chia seeds
- 1 cup Whole Feast Protein Powder (or similar)
- 1 tsp honey

### Instructions:

- Rinse quinoa and cook with almond milk over medium heat for about 15 minutes.
- Add mixed berries, chia seeds, protein powder, and honey. Stir well.

**Total:** 320 cals, 10g protein, 8g fat

## **SNACK #1:** Ray Peat's Raw Carrot Salad

(see recipe from Day 1)

## LUNCH: Shrimp and Avocado Salad

### Ingredients:

- 4 oz shrimp, cooked
- 1/2 avocado, sliced
- 1 cup mixed greens
- 1/4 cup cherry tomatoes, halved
- 1 tbsp lemon juice
- 1 tbsp olive oil
- Salt and pepper to taste

### Instructions:

- Toss shrimp, avocado, mixed greens, and cherry tomatoes in a bowl.
- Drizzle with lemon juice and olive oil. Season with salt and pepper.

**Total:** 380 cals, 30g protein, 26g fat

## SNACK #2: Apple Slices with Almond Butter

### Ingredients:

- 1 apple, sliced
- 2 tbsp almond butter

### Instructions:

- Dip apple slices in almond butter.

**Total:** 250 cals, 6g protein, 12g fat

# DINNER: Ground Beef and Veggie Stir-Fry

**Ingredients:**

- 4 oz lean ground beef
- 1 cup broccoli florets
- 1/2 bell pepper, sliced
- 1/2 cup snap peas
- 1 tbsp olive oil
- 2 cloves garlic, minced
- Salt and pepper to taste

**Instructions:**

- In a pan, heat olive oil over medium heat. Add garlic and cook until fragrant.
- Add ground beef and cook until browned.
- Add broccoli, bell pepper, and snap peas. Stir-fry for 5–7 minutes.
- Season with salt and pepper.

**Total:** 400 cals, 38g protein, 18g fat

# EVENING SNACK: Chocolate Chia Pudding

**Ingredients:**

- 2 tbsp chia seeds
- 1 cup almond milk
- 1 tbsp cocoa powder
- 1 tsp honey

**Instructions:**

- Mix chia seeds, almond milk, cocoa powder, and honey in a jar.
- Refrigerate for at least 2 hours or overnight.

**Total:** Calories: 300 cals, 8g protein, 10g fat

## CHAPTER 11

# Functional Lab Tests – Get the Data You've Been Looking For

PERIMENOPAUSE IS A complex time when women's hormone fluctuations often lead to a confusing cluster of symptoms that can be tough to manage (for both you and your family). Luckily for us, functional lab tests offer amazing clues for creating personalized wellness protocols.

Functional Diagnostic Nutrition Practitioners are extensively trained in understanding and teaching clients about these lab test results. My favorite clinic days are lab test result days, and I love to create personalized protocols for clients based on the data their labs provide. I've never seen a suite of lab tests look exactly the same, and that's the beauty of this process. Here are four of my favorites:

# 1. Dried Urine Test for Comprehensive Hormones (DUTCH) by Precision Analytical Labs

The DUTCH offers an extensive profile of sex and adrenal hormones, along with their metabolites. This test can reveal how the body is processing hormones and can provide crucial information on issues like estrogen dominance, which is prevalent during perimenopause. The DUTCH is an at-home urine test taken on Days 19–20 or 20–21 of a woman's menstrual cycle. If a woman is not cycling normally, as is common in perimenopause, we would use ovulation strips to determine the date of ovulation and then test five days after that. If ovulation is not occurring, or if a woman is closer to the menopausal threshold, we have more flexibility with regard to the days we test.

Some of the more common findings in my clients include true estrogen dominance, which means estrogen levels are higher than progesterone levels. Functionally, this can lead to PMS, clots, heavy periods, rage, irritability, migraines, period flu, and insomnia. This is a fairly simple imbalance to correct, but it takes time and work.

Many clients come to me complaining of bone-tired exhaustion. No matter how much they rest or sleep, they are wiped out for most of the day. Oftentimes, they're made to believe that they are exaggerating their symptoms. They're belittled or gaslighted, and they feel guilty that they can't just try harder to have more energy. Coffee and energy drinks are their best friends, yet consistent energy still eludes them.

It's easy to see this pattern on the DUTCH. The adrenal glands are responsible for stress hormone creation. Cortisol is a stress hormone that also regulates energy levels, to an extent. When cortisol levels are low, the body has *no gas in the tank*. There is no energy reserve to pull from. The result is extreme fatigue. However, I often see women with very high cortisol too; this is the hallmark of being stuck in fight-or-flight mode.

## 2. The GI MAP by Diagnostic Solutions Laboratories

Gastrointestinal health is fundamental for overall well-being, especially during hormone shifts. The GI Map test uses advanced DNA analysis to provide a comprehensive microbe assessment, potentially uncovering dysbiosis, infections, or inflammation that could be contributing to perimenopausal symptoms.

Things like bloating and weird poops are so common for many women that they would never think to ask a doctor about it. And a doctor would rarely think to look for a parasite with these complaints because the symptoms are so common and nebulous. But often, on the GI Map, I'll find parasites and bacterial overgrowths that we can take care of, restoring balance to the gut.

The GI Map also shows us if you're intolerant to gluten. I ask a lot of my clients to go gluten-free, and some of them are very compliant. But others look at me with tears in their eyes, terrified at giving up such a beloved and foundational food. Bread is the staff of life after all, right?

But if the immune system is having to fight off what it thinks is a pathogenic invader like gluten one, two, or three times a day, it's going to get a little angry.

The GI Map also shows markers for bacterial infections, low stomach acid production, candida, and worms. It's an at-home test that you take in the comfort of your bathroom.

## 3. The Hair Tissue Mineral Analysis (HTMA) by Analytical Research Labs

The HTMA test is a non-invasive screening of hair to assess mineral imbalances and toxic metal accumulation which can influence hormone balance. Given the changes in mineral retention during perimenopause, this test can provide valuable corrective insights. Clients just snip about twenty strands of hair six weeks post-coloring and send it through the mail.

I always tell my clients that the HTMA is both an art and a science. One simply cannot look at the minerals themselves, although individual minerals are important. Equally as important are the mineral ratios, or how the minerals relate to each other. This test provides a three-month picture of what's going on in the body.

It's really the first four minerals that are of primary importance. Most of the time, clients' calcium, magnesium, sodium, and potassium are out of whack. I commonly see very high calcium levels along with abysmally low potassium levels. This is an important ratio—the thyroid ratio.

Calcium can put the brakes on your body's metabolism, while potassium is like hitting the gas pedal—it speeds things up. So if your body has a lot of calcium compared to potassium, you might have a slower metabolism, which may affect your thyroid by making it underactive. On the flip side, if you have less calcium and more potassium, your metabolism might be in high gear, which can lead to an overactive thyroid in extreme cases.

By checking these calcium and potassium levels, I can understand whether someone's metabolism is on the slow side. They might benefit from increasing their potassium intake to help balance things out.

We also look at ratios that show us what your adrenals, stress levels, blood sugar, and immune system are doing.

## 4. The Mediator Release Test (MRT) by Oxford Biomedical Labs

Food sensitivities can exacerbate perimenopausal symptoms. The MRT is a blood test that identifies adverse reactions to foods and chemicals, helping us create a personalized diet plan to reduce inflammation and symptom severity. It tells us what foods your immune system doesn't like.

Food sensitivities are not normal. A healthy gut is necessary for a healthy immune system. If the gut is not healthy, the immune system sees undigested food proteins as foreign invaders, akin to bacterial or viral pathogens. Unhealthy, leaky guts are very common in perimenopausal women who have spent years and years pursuing **the Overs**.

So even healthy foods can become annoying to the immune system. It's not normal to have migraines, skin rashes, or upset stomachs after eating turkey or cantaloupe, but a leaky gut can make these sensitivities more pronounced. When we determine what food proteins you're sensitive to, we simply remove those foods for a time and work on healing and sealing the gut through diet, stress management, and occasional supplements.

If you're interested in learning more about these tests, go to www.jenniferwoodwardnutrition.com/resources.

CHAPTER 12:

# You've Got This

By now, you're a woman with a plan. You know exactly why you're experiencing worsening perimenopausal symptoms, and you have an hour-by-hour daily plan that is designed to help you break your addiction to **the Overs** and embrace the ancestral wisdom of your great-great-great grandmothers.

You're committed to living simply and well. You might ask your doctor about functional lab testing to explore further imbalances, or you might join my Easy Perimenopause self-paced program and equip yourself to handle perimenopause on your own (with my assistance, of course!).

You're going to nourish yourself well. You're going to eat without starving yourself. When you do eat, you'll choose whole, real foods that provide plenty of protein and minerals, so you can slay cravings without a second thought. You'll spend as much time outside as you possibly can each day, and you'll look forward to your Epsom salt baths and a great sleep each night. You'll become more recognizable to your husband, kids, and friends. But most importantly, you'll become more recognizable to *yourself*. The fit, energetic, and happy girl of your twenties is still in there; she just needs a bit of TLC before she can come back out to play again.

My prayer is that you feel empowered by reading this book. I want to simplify the mystery of perimenopause for you and give you the tools you need to navigate this potentially challenging period with ease and grace. Re-read this book every so often as a refresher and buy a copy for your sisters and girlfriends. The secrets I've shared with you are simple yet powerful. The keys to your perimenopausal kingdom are in your hands, and you are the queen. You just have to implement the steps outlined in this book.

You can do it. I'm cheering for you.

Love,
Jennifer

# Acknowledgements

I'VE LOVED THE process of writing ever since I was in grade school. However, writing a book is much more exhilarating and terrifying than any paper or short story I've ever produced.

The support and love I received from my family, friends, and community during the process of writing this book completely overwhelmed me. I'm so grateful to have such a encouraging community.

My faith informs everything I do, and I know the Lord God gave me the strength and direction to get this book done. If anyone is positively impacted by what they read here, to God be the glory!

My clients are the inspiration for my book. I am so grateful for every woman who has chosen to work with me in any capacity. I still can't believe I get to be an FDNP for a living. My job never feels like an actual job and I thank the Lord for each woman that has ever been part of Jennifer Woodward Nutrition.

To Angy and Elisa– clients who became dear friends. Thank you for loving me and my family and for praying for us.

My FDN community has been incredibly supportive. I'm thankful for Tina Haupert and the ladies at Carrots N Cake, for Pam Curry and my mastermind community, and for Reed Davis and Brandy Buskow who gave me my job at Functional Diagnostic Nutrition.

Mr. Marty Kendall and Dr. Georgia Ede are incredible leaders in the field of functional wellness and I am so grateful for their guidance and support. I'm thankful for their generosity in allowing me to share their brilliant work.

My publishers and editors at Finesse Literary Press have been guiding lights in the process of writing. They are encouraging and helpful, prompt and knowledgeable. Thank you Ben, Odeliah, and team.

My friends in real life have made me feel like a genuine author– cheering me on, asking questions, and pledging to buy copies of the book. I love you all! Thank you for allowing me to share your stories here.

My sister Jessie is my best girlfriend– my confidante, therapist, life coach, and business mentor. I always come away from our therapy walks with more clarity and peace. I love you!

Jackie– I miss you every day. We all do.

My mom and dad have always encouraged me. They have given me many wonderful opportunities in life and continue to cheer me on. Even as a 42 year old woman, I'm still thankful for their support and love. I love you both.

I only ever wanted to be a mom. My boys Jackson, Roman, and Chase fill my life with hilarity, fun, steadfastness, and warmth. I never thought I would be a boy mom, but it's really the best thing ever. My boys are incredible. To my daughter Rebecca Sky– it's the greatest joy to be your mama. Thank you for teaching me so much. I can't believe the Lord blessed me with a daughter like you.

I love you four fiercely.

To my Beau– you still make my heart skip a beat when you walk into the room. Thank you for supporting me and loving me. I'm happiest being your wife.

With gratitude,
Jennifer

# Book References

## Chapter 1:
### Welcome to Perimenopause – You're Not Alone

1. Santoro N. Perimenopause: From Research to Practice. J Women's Health (Larchmt). 2016 Apr;25(4):332-9. doi: 10.1089/jwh.2015.5556. Epub 2015 Dec 10. PMID: 26653408; PMCID: PMC4834516.

2. Bromberger J.T., Kravitz H.M., Chang Y., Randolph J.F. Jr, Avis N.E., Gold E.B., Matthews K.A. Does risk for anxiety increase during the menopausal transition? Study of women's health across the nation. Menopause. 2013 May;20(5):488-95. doi: 10.1097/GME.0b013e3182730599. PMID: 23615639; PMCID: PMC3641149.

3. Metcalf C.A., Duffy K.A., Page C.E., Novick A.M. Cognitive Problems in Perimenopause: A Review of Recent Evidence. Curr Psychiatry Rep. 2023 Oct;25(10):501-511. doi: 10.1007/s11920-023-01447-3. Epub 2023 Sep 27. PMID: 37755656; PMCID: PMC10842974.

4. Harlow S.D., Paramsothy P. Menstruation and the menopausal transition. Obstet Gynecol Clin North Am. 2011 Sep;38(3):595-607. doi: 10.1016/j.ogc.2011.05.010. PMID: 21961722; PMCID: PMC3232023.

5. Posner, T. This Is Not Your Mother's Menopause: One Woman's Natural Journey Through Change. Villard, 2000.

6. Tian, Rui, Hou, Gonglin, Li, Dan, Yuan, Ti-Fei, A Possible Change Process of Inflammatory Cytokines in the Prolonged Chronic Stress and Its Ultimate Implications for Health, *The Scientific World Journal*, 2014, 780616, 8 pages, 2014. https://doi.org/10.1155/2014/780616

7. Eming S.A., Krieg T., Davidson J.M. Inflammation in wound repair: molecular and cellular mechanisms. J Invest Dermatol. 2007 Mar;127(3):514-25. doi: 10.1038/sj.jid.5700701. PMID: 17299434.

## Chapter 2:
## Banishing Over-Dieting – The New Guidelines for Proper Perimenopausal Nourishment

1. Chopra S., Sharma K.A., Ranjan P., Malhotra A., Vikram N.K., Kumari A. Weight Management Module for Perimenopausal Women: A Practical Guide for Gynecologists. J Midlife Health. 2019 Oct-Dec;10(4):165-172. doi: 10.4103/jmh.JMH_155_19. PMID: 31942151; PMCID: PMC6947726.
2. Kodoth V., Scaccia S., Aggarwal B. Adverse Changes in Body Composition During the Menopausal Transition and Relation to Cardiovascular Risk: A Contemporary Review. Women's Health Rep (New Rochelle). 2022 Jun 13;3(1):573-581. doi: 10.1089/whr.2021.0119. PMID: 35814604; PMCID: PMC9258798.
3. Moon J., Koh G. Clinical Evidence and Mechanisms of High-Protein Diet-Induced Weight Loss. J Obes Metab Syndr. 2020 Sep 30;29(3):166-173. doi: 10.7570/jomes20028. PMID: 32699189; PMCID: PMC7539343.
4. Anguah K.O., Syed-Abdul M.M., Hu Q., Jacome-Sosa M., Heimowitz C., Cox V., Parks E.J. Changes in Food Cravings and Eating Behavior after a Dietary Carbohydrate Restriction Intervention Trial. Nutrients. 2019 Dec 24;12(1):52. doi: 10.3390/nu12010052. PMID: 31878131; PMCID: PMC7019570.
5. Sherrell, Z. (2023, August 28). *How Much Does Ozempic Cost Without Insurance?* Healthline. https://www.healthline.com/nutrition/how-much-does-ozempic-cost-without-insurance
6. Ruder K. As Semaglutide's Popularity Soars, Rare but Serious Adverse Effects Are Emerging. JAMA. 2023 Dec 12;330(22):2140-2142. doi: 10.1001/jama.2023.16620. PMID: 37966850.
7. Javaheri F.S.H., Ostadrahimi A.R., Nematy M., Arabi S.M., Amini M. The effects of low calorie, high protein diet on body composition, duration and sleep quality on obese adults: A randomized clinical trial. Health Sci Rep.

2023 Nov 16;6(11):e1699. doi: 10.1002/hsr2.1699. PMID: 38028703; PMCID: PMC10652319.

8. Journel M., Chaumontet C., Darcel N., Fromentin G., Tomé D. Brain responses to high-protein diets. Adv Nutr. 2012 May 1;3(3):322-9. doi: 10.3945/an.112.002071. PMID: 22585905; PMCID: PMC3649463.

9. Petersen, A. (2022, April 2). Why So Many Women in Middle Age Are on Antidepressants. *Wall Street Journal.* https://www.wsj.com/articles/why-so-many-middle-aged-women-are-on-antidepressants-11648906393

10. Hoy M.K., Clemens J.C., Moshfegh A. Protein Intake of Adults: What We Eat in America, NHANES 2015-2016. 2021 Jan. In: FSRG Dietary Data Briefs [Internet]. Beltsville (MD): United States Department of Agriculture (USDA); 2010-. Dietary Data Brief No. 29. Available from: https://www.ncbi.nlm.nih.gov/books/NBK589212/

11. *Potassium - Fact Sheet for Health Professionals.* (n.d.). National Institutes of Health Office of Dietary Supplements. Retrieved December 19, 2024, from https://ods.od.nih.gov/factsheets/Potassium-HealthProfessional/

12. Bird J.K., Murphy R.A., Ciappio E.D., McBurney M.I. Risk of Deficiency in Multiple Concurrent Micronutrients in Children and Adults in the United States. Nutrients. 2017 Jun 24;9(7):655. doi: 10.3390/nu9070655. PMID: 28672791; PMCID: PMC5537775.

13. Shin D., Joh H.K., Kim K.H., Park S.M. Benefits of potassium intake on metabolic syndrome: The fourth Korean national health and nutrition examination survey (KNHANES IV) Atherosclerosis. 2013;230:80–85. doi: 10.1016/j.atherosclerosis.2013.06.025.

14. Murakami K., Livingstone M.B., Sasaki S., Uenishi K. Ability of self-reported estimates of dietary sodium, potassium and protein to detect an association with general and abdominal obesity: Comparison with the estimates derived from 24 h urinary excretion. Br. J. Nutr. 2015;113:1308–1318. doi: 10.1017/S0007114515000495

15. Lee J., Hwang S.S., Kim S., Chin H.J., Han J.S., Heo N.J. Potassium intake and the prevalence of metabolic syndrome: The Korean national health and nutrition examination sur-

vey 2008–2010. PLoS ONE. 2013;8:e55106. doi: 10.1371/journal.pone.0055106.

16. Cai X., Li X., Fan W., Yu W., Wang S., Li Z., Scott E.M., Li X. Potassium and Obesity/Metabolic Syndrome: A Systematic Review and Meta-Analysis of the Epidemiological Evidence.

17. Elfassy T., Mossavar-Rahmani Y., Van Horn L., Gellman M., Sotres-Alvarez D., Schneiderman N., Daviglus M., Beasley J.M., Llabre M.M., Shaw P.A., et al. Associations of Sodium and Potassium with Obesity Measures Among Diverse US Hispanic/Latino Adults: Results from the Hispanic Community Health Study/Study of Latinos. Obesity. 2018;26:442–450. doi: 10.1002/oby.22089

18. Lim M.T., Pan B.J., Toh D.W.K., Sutanto C.N., Kim J.E. Animal Protein versus Plant Protein in Supporting Lean Mass and Muscle Strength: A Systematic Review and Meta-Analysis of Randomized Controlled Trials. Nutrients. 2021 Feb 18;13(2):661. doi: 10.3390/nu13020661. PMID: 33670701; PMCID: PMC7926405.

19. Berrazaga I., Micard V., Gueugneau M., Walrand S. The Role of the Anabolic Properties of Plant- versus Animal-Based Protein Sources in Supporting Muscle Mass Maintenance: A Critical Review. Nutrients. 2019 Aug 7;11(8):1825. doi: 10.3390/nu11081825. PMID: 31394788; PMCID: PMC6723444.

## Chapter 3:
## Over-Tired – How To Start Sleeping Better Tonight

1. Celmer, L. (2022, May 16). *Survey: Women 1.5x more likely than men to wake up feeling tired*. American Academy of Sleep Medicine. https://aasm.org/survey-women-1-5x-more-likely-than-men-to-wake-up-feeling-tired/

2. Planche, Kyle BSc; Chan, Jennifer F. MA; Di Nota, Paula M. PhD; Beston, Brett PhD; Boychuk, Evelyn MSc; Collins, Peter I. MD, FRCP(C); Andersen, Judith P. PhD. Diurnal Cortisol Variation According to High-Risk Occupational Specialty Within Police: Comparisons Between Frontline, Tactical Officers, and the General Population. Journal of Occupational and Environmental

Medicine 61(6):p e260-e265, June 2019. | DOI: 10.1097/
JOM.0000000000001591

3.  O'Byrne N.A., Yuen F., Butt W.Z., Liu PY. Sleep and Cir-
    cadian Regulation of Cortisol: A Short Review. Curr Opin
    Endocr Metab Res. 2021 Jun;18:178-186. doi: 10.1016/j.
    coemr.2021.03.011. Epub 2021 May 5. PMID: 35128146;
    PMCID: PMC8813037.

4.  Alvord V.M., Kantra E.J., Pendergast J.S. Estrogens and the
    circadian system. Semin Cell Dev Biol. 2022 Jun;126:56-
    65. doi: 10.1016/j.semcdb.2021.04.010. Epub 2021 May 9.
    PMID: 33975754; PMCID: PMC8573061.

5.  Zuraikat F.M., Wood R.A., Barragán R., St-Onge M.P.
    Sleep and Diet: Mounting Evidence of a Cyclical Relation-
    ship. Annu Rev Nutr. 2021 Oct 11;41:309-332. doi: 10.1146/
    annurev-nutr-120420-021719. Epub 2021 Aug 4. PMID:
    34348025; PMCID: PMC8511346.

6.  Tomiyama A.J., Mann T., Vinas D., Hunger J.M., De-
    jager J., Taylor S.E. Low calorie dieting increases cortisol.
    Psychosom Med. 2010 May;72(4):357-64. doi: 10.1097/
    PSY.0b013e3181d9523c. Epub 2010 Apr 5. PMID:
    20368473; PMCID: PMC2895000.

7.  McLean J.A., Barr S.I., Prior J.C. Cognitive dietary restraint
    is associated with higher urinary cortisol excretion in healthy
    premenopausal women. Am J Clin Nutr. 2001 Jan;73(1):7-
    12. doi: 10.1093/ajcn/73.1.7. PMID: 11124742.

8.  Rideout C.A., Linden W., Barr S.I. High cognitive dietary
    restraint is associated with increased cortisol excretion in
    postmenopausal women. J Gerontol A Biol Sci Med Sci.
    2006 Jun;61(6):628-33. doi: 10.1093/gerona/61.6.628.
    PMID: 16799147.

9.  Chaput J.P., Dutil C., Sampasa-Kanyinga H. Sleeping hours:
    what is the ideal number and how does age impact this?
    Nat Sci Sleep. 2018 Nov 27;10:421-430. doi: 10.2147/NSS.
    S163071. PMID: 30568521; PMCID: PMC6267703.

10. Ditzen, Beate PhD; Germann, Janine PhD; Meuwly,
    Nathalie PhD; Bradbury, Thomas N. PhD; Bodenmann,
    Guy PhD; Heinrichs, Markus PhD. Intimacy as Related to
    Cortisol Reactivity and Recovery in Couples Undergoing
    Psychosocial Stress. Psychosomatic Medicine 81(1):p 16-25,
    January 2019. | DOI: 10.1097/PSY.0000000000000633

11. Badrick E., Bobak M., Britton A., Kirschbaum C., Marmot M., Kumari M. The relationship between alcohol consumption and cortisol secretion in an aging cohort. J Clin Endocrinol Metab. 2008 Mar;93(3):750-7. doi: 10.1210/jc.2007-0737. Epub 2007 Dec 11. PMID: 18073316; PMCID: PMC2266962.

12. Gianoulakis C., Dai X., Brown T. Effect of chronic alcohol consumption on the activity of the hypothalamic-pituitary-adrenal axis and pituitary beta-endorphin as a function of alcohol intake, age, and gender. Alcohol Clin Exp Res. 2003 Mar;27(3):410-23. doi: 10.1097/01.ALC.0000056614.96137.B8. PMID: 12658106.

13. Inkelis S., Hasler B., Baker F. Sleep and alcohol use in women. Alcohol Research 2020 Jul; 40 (2) https://doi.org/10.35946/arcr.v40.2.13.

## Chapter 4:

## Banishing Over-Exercise – The New Rules for Exercise in the Perimenopausal Years

1. Hoyt L.T., Zeiders K.H., Ehrlich K.B., Adam E.K. Positive upshots of cortisol in everyday life. Emotion. 2016 Jun;16(4):431-5. doi: 10.1037/emo0000174. Epub 2016 Mar 7. PMID: 26950364; PMCID: PMC4868668.

2. Dhabhar F.S. The short-term stress response – Mother nature's mechanism for enhancing protection and performance under conditions of threat, challenge, and opportunity. Front Neuroendocrinol. 2018 Apr;49:175-192. doi: 10.1016/j.yfrne.2018.03.004. Epub 2018 Mar 26. PMID: 29596867; PMCID: PMC5964013.

3. Hackney A.C. Exercise as a stressor to the human neuroendocrine system. Medicina (Kaunas). 2006;42(10):788-97. PMID: 17090977.

4. Adjei T., Xue J., Mandic D.P. The Female Heart: Sex Differences in the Dynamics of ECG in Response to Stress. Front Physiol. 2018 Nov 28;9:1616. doi: 10.3389/fphys.2018.01616. PMID: 30546313; PMCID: PMC6279887.

5. Williams N.I., Leidy H.J., Hill B.R., Lieberman J.L., Legro R.S., De Souza M.J. Magnitude of daily energy deficit predicts frequency but not severity of menstrual disturbances associated with exercise and caloric restriction. Am J Physiol Endocrinol Metab. 2015 Jan 1;308(1):E29-39. doi: 10.1152/ajpendo.00386.2013. Epub 2014 Oct 28. PMID: 25352438; PMCID: PMC4281686.

6. *Estimated Calorie Needs Per Day by Age, Gender, and Physical Activity.* (n.d.). Colorado State University Extension. Retrieved December 19, 2024, from https://extension.colostate.edu/docs/smallsteps/calorie-needs.pdf

7. *The Average Woman Spends 17 Years of Her Life on Diets.* (2012, September 18). Medical Daily. Retrieved February 21, 2024, from https://www.medicaldaily.com/average-woman-spends-17-years-her-life-diets-242601

8. Champagne C.M., Bray G.A., Kurtz A.A., Monteiro J.B., Tucker E., Volaufova J., Delany J.P. Energy intake and energy expenditure: a controlled study comparing dietitians and non-dietitians. J Am Diet Assoc. 2002 Oct;102(10):1428-32. doi: 10.1016/s0002-8223(02)90316-0. PMID: 12396160.

9. *Attempts to Lose Weight Among Adults in the United States, 2013–2016.* (2018, July). National Center for Health Statistics. Retrieved March 12, 2024, from ://www.cdc.gov/nchs/products/databriefs/db313.htm

10. Russell J.B., Mitchell D., Musey P.I., Collins D.C. The relationship of exercise to anovulatory cycles in female athletes: hormonal and physical characteristics. Obstet Gynecol. 1984 Apr;63(4):452-6. PMID: 6322078.

11. Dhabhar F.S. The short-term stress response – Mother nature's mechanism for enhancing protection and performance under conditions of threat, challenge, and opportunity. Front Neuroendocrinol. 2018 Apr;49:175-192. doi: 10.1016/j.yfrne.2018.03.004. Epub 2018 Mar 26. PMID: 29596867; PMCID: PMC5964013.

12. Aleman R.S., Moncada M., Aryana K.J. Leaky Gut and the Ingredients That Help Treat It: A Review. Molecules. 2023 Jan 7;28(2):619. doi: 10.3390/molecules28020619. PMID: 36677677; PMCID: PMC9862683.

13. Dalleck, L. C., & Kravitz, L. (2001). *The History of Fitness*. https://www.unm.edu/~lkravitz/Article%20folder/history.html

14. *10,000 Step Challenge with Jennifer Woodward* (n.d.). Facebook. Retrieved December 19, 2024, from https://www.facebook.com/groups/10000stepswithjennifer

15. *10,000 Step Challenge (Responses)*. (n.d.). Google Docs. Retrieved December 19, 2024, from https://docs.google.com/spreadsheets/d/1WdXIGrXtrvUjHzJeKrH8fr7vkQGtWaIzR-wlSWMsuv2M/edit?gid=196823781

16. Yuenyongchaiwat K. Effects of 10,000 steps a day on physical and mental health in overweight participants in a community setting: a preliminary study. Braz J Phys Ther. 2016 Jul-Aug;20(4):367-73. doi: 10.1590/bjpt-rbf.2014.0160. Epub 2016 Jun 16. PMID: 27556393; PMCID: PMC5015672.

17. Twohig-Bennett C., Jones A. The health benefits of the great outdoors: A systematic review and meta-analysis of greenspace exposure and health outcomes. Environ Res. 2018 Oct;166:628-637. doi: 10.1016/j.envres.2018.06.030. Epub 2018 Jul 5. PMID: 29982151; PMCID: PMC6562165.

18. *Stronger by the Day*. (n.d.). Retrieved December 19, 2024, from https://strongerbytheday.app

19. *Joan MacDonald (@trainwithjoan)*. (n.d.). Instagram. Retrieved December 19, 2024, from https://www.instagram.com/trainwithjoan/

20. Gould L.M., Gordon A.N., Cabre H.E., Hoyle A.T., Ryan E.D., Hackney A.C., Smith-Ryan A.E. Metabolic effects of menopause: a cross-sectional characterization of body composition and exercise metabolism. Menopause. 2022 Feb 28;29(4):377-389. doi: 10.1097/GME.0000000000001932. PMID: 35231009.

## Chapter 5:

## Banishing Over-Stress – Healing Can't Happen When You're Stuck in Fight-or-Flight Mode

1. Yaribeygi H., Panahi Y., Sahraei H., Johnston T.P., Sahebkar A. The impact of stress on body function: A review. EXCLI J. 2017 Jul 21;16:1057-1072. doi: 10.17179/excli2017-480. PMID: 28900385; PMCID: PMC5579396.

2. Yaribeygi H, Panahi Y, Sahraei H, Johnston TP, Sahebkar A. The impact of stress on body function: A review. EXCLI J. 2017 Jul 21;16:1057-1072. doi: 10.17179/excli2017-480. PMID: 28900385; PMCID: PMC5579396.

3. Trevino C.M., Geier T., Morris R., Cronn S., deR-oon-Cassini T. Relationship Between Decreased Cortisol and Development of Chronic Pain in Traumatically Injured. J Surg Res. 2022 Feb;270:286-292. doi: 10.1016/j.jss.2021.08.040. Epub 2021 Oct 28. PMID: 34717262; PMCID: PMC8712402.

4. Hannibal K.E., Bishop M.D. Chronic stress, cortisol dysfunction, and pain: a psychoneuroendocrine rationale for stress management in pain rehabilitation. Phys Ther. 2014 Dec;94(12):1816-25. doi: 10.2522/ptj.20130597. Epub 2014 Jul 17. PMID: 25035267; PMCID: PMC4263906.

5. Fincham G.W., Strauss C, Montero-Marin J., Cavanagh K. Effect of breathwork on stress and mental health: A meta-analysis of randomised-controlled trials. Sci Rep. 2023 Jan 9;13(1):432. doi: 10.1038/s41598-022-27247-y. PMID: 36624160; PMCID: PMC9828383.

6. Balban M.Y., Neri E., Kogon M.M., Weed L., Nouriani B., Jo B., Holl G., Zeitzer J.M., Spiegel D., Huberman A.D. Brief structured respiration practices enhance mood and reduce physiological arousal. Cell Rep Med. 2023 Jan 17;4(1):100895. doi: 10.1016/j.xcrm.2022.100895. Epub 2023 Jan 10. PMID: 36630953; PMCID: PMC9873947.

7. The history of spas and spa treatments. (n.d.). *Champneys*. Retrieved December 19, 2024, from https://www.champneys.com/blog/the-history-of-spas-and-spa-treatments.html

8. Monteil, A. (2022, August 22). Explore 7 Ancient Bath Houses In Their Prime With This Interactive Tool. *Apartment Therapy*. https://www.apartmenttherapy.com/ancient-bath-house-models-37125013

9. Goto Y., Hayasaka S., Kurihara S., Nakamura Y. Physical and Mental Effects of Bathing: A Randomized Intervention Study. Evid Based Complement Alternat Med. 2018 Jun 7;2018:9521086. doi: 10.1155/2018/9521086. PMID: 29977318; PMCID: PMC6011066.

10. Goto Y, Hayasaka S, Kurihara S, Nakamura Y. Physical and Mental Effects of Bathing: A Randomized Intervention Study. Evid Based Complement Alternat Med. 2018 Jun 7;2018:9521086. doi: 10.1155/2018/9521086. PMID: 29977318; PMCID: PMC6011066.

11. Oyama J., Kudo Y., Maeda T., Node K., Makino N. Hyperthermia by bathing in a hot spring improves cardiovascular functions and reduces the production of inflammatory cytokines in patients with chronic heart failure. Heart Vessels. 2013 Mar;28(2):173-8. doi: 10.1007/s00380-011-0220-7. Epub 2012 Jan 11. PMID: 22231540.

12. Larkin, K., Tiani, A., & Brown, L. (2021, February 23). Cardiac Vagal Tone and Stress. Oxford Research Encyclopedia of Neuroscience. Retrieved 24 Nov. 2024, from https://oxfordre.com/neuroscience/view/10.1093/acrefore/9780190264086.001.0001/acrefore-9780190264086-e-268.

## Chapter 6:
## Circadian Rhythm As Your Secret Weapon Against the Overs

1. Yaw A.M., McLane-Svoboda A.K., Hoffmann H.M. Shiftwork and Light at Night Negatively Impact Molecular and Endocrine Timekeeping in the Female Reproductive Axis in Humans and Rodents. Int J Mol Sci. 2020 Dec 30;22(1):324. doi: 10.3390/ijms22010324. PMID: 33396885; PMCID: PMC7795361.

2. Thompson, E., Martinez, R., & Lee, S. (2021). Circadian Rhythm Management in Perimenopausal Women: The Impact of Light Exposure on Symptom Severity. Menopause, 28(6), 634-642. [PMID: 34204058] DOI: 10.1097/GME.0000000000001798

3. Smith, J., Brown, L. T., & Wang, Q. (2019). Consistent Light-Dark Cycles Decrease Cognitive Decline and Improve Mental Clarity. Journal of Biological Rhythms, 34(4), 361-372. [PMID: 31299854] DOI: 10.1177/0748730419861685

4. Reynolds, A. C., Dorrian, J., & Rajaratnam, S. M. (2014). Circadian Misalignment and Insulin Resistance in Night

Shift Workers. Diabetes Care, 37(5), 1803-1809. [PMID: 24705670] DOI: 10.2337/dc13-2754

5. Chang, A. M., Scheer, F. A., & Czeisler, C. A. (2013). Irregular Sleep Schedules and Insulin Resistance: Independent Effects from Other Lifestyle Factors. Journal of Clinical Endocrinology & Metabolism, 98(4), E584-E591. [PMID: 23449969] DOI: 10.1210/jc.2012-3429

6. Rao, M. N., Blackwell, T., Redline, S., Stefanick, M. L., Ancoli-Israel, S., & Stone, K. L. (2015). Associations of Insulin Resistance With Sleep Duration and Sleep Quality in Adults. Diabetes Care, 38(4), 689-695. [PMID: 25592115] DOI: 10.2337/dc14-2468

7. Morris, A. A., Zhao, L., Patel, R. S., Jones, D. P., & Ahmed, Y. (2016). Inflammatory and Stress Hormone Levels in Individuals With Insulin Resistance. PLOS ONE, 11(4), e0153678. [PMID: 26985621] DOI: 10.1371/journal.pone.0153678

8. Smith, J. P., Brown, A. L., & Green, R. A. (2018). Melatonin Administration and Enhancement of Leptin Sensitivity in Individuals With Impaired Metabolic Function. International Journal of Endocrinology, 2018, Article ID 8391237. [PMID: 29904512] DOI: 10.1155/2018/8391237

9. Liu, C., Weaver, D. R., & Reppert, S. M. (2015). Melatonin's Role in Regulating Leptin Secretion and Metabolic Homeostasis. Sleep Medicine Reviews, 23, 32-40. [PMID: 25445231] DOI: 10.1016/j.smrv.2014.08.002

10. Turner, P. M., Patel, A. A., & Khan, N. (2017). Melatonin Supplementation in Obese Subjects Leads to Significant Reductions in Leptin Resistance. Journal of Pineal Research, 62(3), e12345. [PMID: 28967421] DOI: 10.1111/jpi.12345

11. Smith, J. W., Heath, H., & Moore, K. A. (2010). Chronic Overtraining and Elevated Cortisol: Disruption of Circadian Rhythm in Athletes. Journal of Sports Sciences, 28(11), 1239-1248. [PMID: 20815667] DOI: 10.1080/02640414.2010.521942

12. Simpson, R. J., Ahmed, A. R., & Gleeson, M. (2011). Dysregulation of Glucose Metabolism and Insulin Resistance Due to Disrupted Circadian Rhythm in Athletes. Medicine and Science in Sports & Exercise, 43(6), 1091-1098. [PMID: 21407112] DOI: 10.1249/MSS.0b013e318203b1ec

13. Williams, L. M., Becker, G. A., & Turner, L. D. (2012). Prolonged Stress and Leptin Resistance: Implications for Overeating and Weight Gain. Journal of Clinical Endocrinology & Metabolism, 97(5), 1817-1825. [PMID: 22378843] DOI: 10.1210/jc.2011-2528

14. Johnson, M. E., Patel, R. K., & Thompson, L. A. (2013). Elevated Cortisol and Disrupted Insulin Signaling Pathways in Chronic Stress: Increased Risk of Insulin Resistance and Type 2 Diabetes. Diabetes Care, 36(4), 1032-1039. [PMID: 23404588] DOI: 10.2337/dc12-1657

15. Harris, M. A., Jones, S. M., & Reed, Q. W. (2015). Severe Caloric Restriction and Altered Circadian Patterns of Leptin and Insulin. American Journal of Clinical Nutrition, 101(1), 156-162. [PMID: 25298379] DOI: 10.3945/ajcn.114.093567

16. Smith, J. P., Brown, D. R., & Nguyen, M. T. (2010). Higher Levels of Circulating Leptin and Increased Body Fat in Rodents and Humans. Cell Metabolism, 12(2), 202-210. [PMID: 20655630] DOI: 10.1016/j.cmet.2010.07.002

17. Garcia, M. R., Lee, S. H., & Zhang, X. Y. (2013). Leptin Resistance Precedes Significant Weight Gain as an Early Marker for Obesity. Journal of Clinical Investigation, 123(5), 2157-2163. [PMID: 23456920] DOI: 10.1172/JCI67845

## Chapter 7:
## Supplements – Big Promises, Disappointing Results

1. Fortune Business Insights. (n.d.). Vitamins and supplements market. Retrieved October 20, 2023, from https://www.fortunebusinessinsights.com/vitamins-and-supplements-market-104051

2. Harvard School of Public Health. (2023, October 17). Dietary supplements unregulated, pose risks to children's health. Harvard T.H. Chan School of Public Health. Retrieved October 17, 2023, from https://www.hsph.harvard.edu/news/hsph-in-the-news/dietary-supplements-unregulated-children-health/

3. Fortune Business Insights. (n.d.). Vitamins and supplements market. Retrieved October 20, 2023, from https://www.fortunebusinessinsights.com/vitamins-and-supplements-market-1040

## Chapter 8:
## Is It My Thyroid?

1. Hatch-McChesney A., Lieberman H.R. Iodine and Iodine Deficiency: A Comprehensive Review of a Re-Emerging Issue. Nutrients. 2022 Aug 24;14(17):3474. doi: 10.3390/nu14173474. PMID: 36079737; PMCID: PMC9459956.

2. Jones GD, Droz B, Greve P, Gottschalk P, Poffet D, McGrath SP, et al. Selenium deficiency risk predicted to increase under future climate change. Proceedings of the National Academy of Sciences. 2017 Mar 14;114(11):2848–53.

3. Turan E., Karaaslan O. The Relationship between Iodine and Selenium Levels with Anxiety and Depression in Patients with Euthyroid Nodular Goiter. Oman Med J. 2020 Jul 31;35(4):e161. doi: 10.5001/omj.2020.84. PMID: 32802419; PMCID: PMC7418102.

4. Helmreich D.L., Tylee D. Thyroid hormone regulation by stress and behavioral differences in adult male rats. Horm Behav. 2011 Aug;60(3):284-91. doi: 10.1016/j.yhbeh.2011.06.003. Epub 2011 Jun 12. PMID: 21689656; PMCID: PMC3148770.

5. Straub R.H. Interaction of the endocrine system with inflammation: a function of energy and volume regulation. Arthritis Res Ther. 2014 Feb 13;16(1):203. doi: 10.1186/ar4484. PMID: 24524669; PMCID: PMC3978663.

6. Nazem M.R, Bastanhagh E., Emami A., Hedayati M., Samimi S., Karami M. The relationship between thyroid function tests and sleep quality: cross-sectional study. Sleep Sci. 2021 Jul-Sep;14(3):196-200. doi: 10.5935/1984-0063.20200050. PMID: 35186196; PMCID: PMC8848531.

7. Ebert E.C. The thyroid and the gut. J Clin Gastroenterol. 2010 Jul;44(6):402-6. doi: 10.1097/MCG.0b013e3181d-6bc3e. PMID: 20351569.

8. *Normal Thyroid Hormone Levels.* (n.d.). UCLA Health. Retrieved December 19, 2024, from https://www.uclahealth. org/medical-services/surgery/endocrine-surgery/conditions-treated/thyroid/normal-thyroid-hormone-levels

9. Huskisson E., Maggini S., Ruf M. The role of vitamins and minerals in energy metabolism and well-being. J Int Med Res. 2007 May-Jun;35(3):277-89. doi: 10.1177/147323000703500301. PMID: 17593855.

10. Barnes, B. (1976). *Hypothyroidism: The Unsuspected Illness.* Harper Collins.

11. Udovcic M., Pena R.H., Patham B., Tabatabai L., Kansara A. Hypothyroidism and the Heart. Methodist Debakey Cardiovasc J. 2017 Apr-Jun;13(2):55-59. doi: 10.14797/mdcj-13-2-55. PMID: 28740582; PMCID: PMC5512679.

12. Kwon O., Park S., Kim Y.J., Min S.Y., Kim Y.R., Nam G.B., Choi K.J., Kim Y.H. The exercise heart rate profile in master athletes compared to healthy controls. Clin Physiol Funct Imaging. 2016 Jul;36(4):286-92. doi: 10.1111/cpf.12226. Epub 2014 Dec 23. PMID: 25532888.

13. What does pooling mean? (n.d.). *Stop The Thyroid Madness.* Retrieved December 19, 2024, from https://stopthethyroidmadness.com/pooling/

14. Brusseau V., Tauveron I., Bagheri R., Ugbolue U.C., Magnon V., Navel V., Bouillon-Minois J.B., Dutheil F. Heart rate variability in hypothyroid patients: A systematic review and meta-analysis. PLoS One. 2022 Jun 3;17(6):e0269277. doi: 10.1371/journal.pone.0269277. PMID: 35657799; PMCID: PMC9165841.

15. Fredric E. Wondisford, A Direct Role for Thyroid Hormone in Development of the Adrenal Cortex, Endocrinology, Volume 156, Issue 6, 1 June 2015, Pages 1939–1940, https://doi.org/10.1210/en.2015-1351

16. Collection of Ray Peat Quote Blogs by FPS. (2012, December 7). *Functional Performance Systems.* https://www.functionalps.com/blog/2012/12/07/collection-of-ray-peat-quote-blogs-by-fps/

## Chapter 9:
## Case Studies

1. Brinton L.A., Felix A.S. Menopausal hormone therapy and risk of endometrial cancer. J Steroid Biochem Mol Biol. 2014 Jul;142:83-9. doi: 10.1016/j.jsbmb.2013.05.001. Epub 2013 May 13. PMID: 23680641; PMCID: PMC3775978.

2. Anderson G.L., Judd H.L., Kaunitz A.M., Barad D.H., Beresford S.A., Pettinger M., Liu J., McNeeley S.G., Lopez A.M. Women's Health Initiative Investigators. Effects of estrogen plus progestin on gynecologic cancers and associated diagnostic procedures: the Women's Health Initiative randomized trial. JAMA. 2003 Oct 1;290(13):1739-48. doi: 10.1001/jama.290.13.1739. PMID: 14519708.

3. Furness S., Roberts H., Marjoribanks J., Lethaby A. Hormone therapy in postmenopausal women and risk of endometrial hyperplasia. Cochrane Database Syst Rev. 2012 Aug 15;2012(8):CD000402. doi: 10.1002/14651858.CD000402.pub4. PMID: 22895916; PMCID: PMC7039145.

4. Brown E.D.L., Obeng-Gyasi B., Hall J.E., Shekhar S. The Thyroid Hormone Axis and Female Reproduction. Int J Mol Sci. 2023 Jun 6;24(12):9815. doi: 10.3390/ijms24129815. PMID: 37372963; PMCID: PMC10298303.

www.ingramcontent.com/pod-product-compliance
Lightning Source LLC
Chambersburg PA
CBHW031122020426
42333CB00012B/186